CAUSAL ANALYSIS
IN BIOMEDICINE
AND EPIDEMIOLOGY

Biostatistics: A Series of References and Textbooks

Series Editor
Shein-Chung Chow

President, U.S. Operations
StatPlus, Inc.
Yardley, Pennsylvania

Adjunct Professor
Temple University
Philadelphia, Pennsylvania

ADDITIONAL VOLUMES IN PREPARATION

CAUSAL ANALYSIS IN BIOMEDICINE AND EPIDEMIOLOGY

BASED ON MINIMAL SUFFICIENT CAUSATION

MIKEL AICKIN

Center for Health Research
Kaiser Permanente Northwest Division
Portland, Oregon

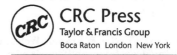

CRC Press
Taylor & Francis Group
Boca Raton London New York

CRC Press is an imprint of the
Taylor & Francis Group, an **informa** business

CRC Press
Taylor & Francis Group
6000 Broken Sound Parkway NW, Suite 300
Boca Raton, FL 33487-2742

First issued in paperback 2019

© 2002 by Taylor & Francis Group, LLC
CRC Press is an imprint of Taylor & Francis Group, an Informa business

No claim to original U.S. Government works

ISBN-13: 978-0-8247-0748-4 (hbk)
ISBN-13: 978-0-367-39674-9 (pbk)

Visit the Taylor & Francis Web site at
http://www.taylorandfrancis.com

and the CRC Press Web site at
http://www.crcpress.com

To CR

Preface

This is a book about the properties of causation. It is based on the idea that even if we do not have a perfect definition of cause, we can nonetheless describe some of its features, and that this will help us to understand its nature. One of the miracles of the human mind is that it can discuss and consider before it understands, and this seems to be where we are at the present time regarding notions of causation.

The book is also about ways in which an understanding of causation can affect how we think about biology, medicine, public health, and epidemiology. As a practicing biostatistician I am all too aware of the degree to which causation is *not* used in the biomedical sciences, and I am reasonably sure that we will progress more rapidly if we overcome our Humean phobia that causation may not be real.

I will admit that there is some mathematics here (mostly a new variant of algebra), but I contend that it is simple, and like most useful mathematics, gives back more in understanding than it extracts in mental sweat. There is some philosophy here, but since I am not a philosopher it is relatively straightforward and blessedly brief. There is also some biomedical science here, either by example or by indirection, because causation is at base a scientific topic. But given all this, I have tried to write this book so that it transcends disciplinary boundaries and speaks to the need we all have to make causation an integral part of our thinking about science, and a natural part of the way we talk about science.

Mikel Aickin

Contents

Special Symbols and Phrases

1

Orientation

The idea of cause-and-effect plays such a constant role in our everyday lives, it is remarkable that after centuries of thought, we still cannot tell whether it is part of the natural order of the universe, or simply a mental construct we use to make sense of what happens to us. Fascinating though this dilemma is, we will not solve it here. What we will do is start with one, particularly simple notion of causation, and then using characteristics that *ought* to be true of cause-and-effect, extend our notion of cause over a very wide variety of situations.

In general, people who write about causation take one of two approaches. They either roll out their own definition or else they mount a campaign to dismember somebody else's. Those who trash the work of others are, I think, the most difficult to read with any degree of sympathy. They pull out the various parts of the victim's definition along with the supporting arguments, and then proceed to develop multiple counter-arguments, from a variety of different and undefined points of view. Since they never allow themselves to be pinned down to what *they* think causation is, we can never tell where their legions of arguments actually come from.

If queried, I suppose such authors would claim that in their minds they have a coherent notion of causation, and all of their arguments are based on that notion. But this assertion is easily skewered by the simple observation that they do not, in fact, demonstrate their coherent notion, and so we are quite free to disbelieve its existence. We might just as well maintain that the only actual idea in their minds is the fantasy that they have a coherent idea of causation, but that in reality they themselves do not know what it is. If this seems a harsh criticism, I recommend that the doubtful reader simply pick up any analytic philosophy journal, or any collection of critical essays on causation, and see whether I am right.

The logical reason that the hyper-critics fail is that it is always possible to destroy any logical theory, if the arguments of destruction are

1

not themselves required to obey the rules of logic. Lewis Carroll became famous by writing stories for children, many parts of which were based on exactly this kind of incoherent deconstructionism.

In the pages that follow, I may occasionally slip into a critical comment about some notion of causation, but I only intend to do this as an aside. It is not my attempt to mount a frontal assault, nor any other kind of attack on any particular notion of causation.

There is, of course, another kind of author, who puts his or her definition out for us to examine. These souls are to be greatly admired for having the courage to attempt, in public, to crack one of the toughest nuts of philosophy. They can be hard to read, however, for a quite different reason. Every philosophical idea of cause has to start somewhere, with some basic definitions, or surrogates for definitions. I maintain that this is exceedingly difficult (and perhaps actually impossible) to do. The consequence is that as we read the unfolding definition, we begin to wonder whether some of the pieces aren't a bit too sweeping in their scope. We are not sure where they might lead, and so we have difficulty accepting the author's confidence that they will ultimately lead somewhere useful. We may be aware of other authors, who in the past have promulgated their definitions with equal confidence, and were then easily shown to be building a philosophy on sand because their fundamental assumptions contained hidden contradictions. It is astonishingly easy to put forward plausible-sounding premises, which are found in the final analysis to contain subtle, unanticipated flaws.

Another difficult point is reached when we think we understand the reasoning behind some part of the definition, but we simply disagree with it. This is a serious problem because it begins to rob us of the intellectual energy to keep the author company down a path that we feel leads to certain oblivion. In fashioning a logical system, one slip, even a small mis-step, can utterly destroy the final work.

My intent here is neither to promulgate my own definition of cause, nor to destroy the definitions of others. I will start with an undefined notion of *sufficient cause*, and then using properties that I believe causation ought to have, I will extend the general notion of cause over a very considerable collection of cases of non-sufficient causation.

I'm going to do this by a *constructive* process. This means that I will require sufficient causation to have some natural properties, and then from these properties I will construct the parts that give the theory more structure and usefulness. If you can't agree that your notion of sufficient cause satisfies these properties, or that my causal properties are reasonable, then you can either read on to see what benefits you would obtain by accepting my conditions, or you can try to re-sell this book to someone more compliant.

One advantage of the constructive approach is that it proceeds by a series of steps, each of which I will make as clear as I can. If in the end you do not agree with me, then you will be able to tell exactly the step at which you disagree. This provides us with a useful place to argue, or failing that, allows us to part with a sense of clarity about why we parted.

To peek ahead, I will first ask that you have a notion of causation that is, at least in some of its applications, *sufficient*. That is, there will be at least some cases in which you are willing to say that when all the components of a cause are present, then the effect happens. Using this and two additional properties, I will use the minimal sufficient cause principle to extend your notion of causation consistently over many situations you may not have considered. I will then show that your notion of causation is related to the special case of *nontrivial implication*, which is a particular causal notion that is very easy to study. Using nontrivial implication I will indicate how observations might shed light on what role various causes might have in producing their effects in your theory.

After this, the remainder of the book will be used to pursue a number of questions that come up fairly naturally, to see how the minimal sufficient cause approach deals with them. My overall aim will be to provide tools that make causal analysis of observations more understandable and powerful.

Here is a thumb-nail sketch of the rest of the book. In the next section *What is Causation?* some historical philosophical issues will be discussed, and my philosophical approach for the purposes of this book laid out. In *Naïve Minimal Sufficient Cause* I will discuss the intuitive notion behind minimal sufficient cause, as it emerged from the pens of the philosopher John Mackie and the epidemiologist Kenneth Rothman. In *Events and Probabilities* I remind the reader about the classical set-up for computing probabilities, but then in *Unitary Algebra* I introduce some novel algebra that fits in extremely well with probability arguments, and turns out to be indispensable for causal models. The first real example of causation is *Nontrivial Implication*, which eventually shows itself to be far more useful than one might think. In order to try to make these abstract ideas concrete, I give some *Tiny Examples* based on some very simple situations.

In *The One-Factor Model* I show how unitary algebra is used to specify a causal probability model, here involving only one cause. As one moves to complex causal systems, graphics becomes almost necessary, and so I introduce some *Graphical Elements* for use in the remainder of the book.

To a great extent the most important section is on *Causations*. Here is where I assume a few properties about a given notion of causation, and then show how to extend that notion using the principles of minimal sufficient cause. Under these simple conditions, all causations have a very strong relationship to nontrivial implication. The last paragraph of this section is crucial to understanding the assumptions in force for the remainder of the book.

A key fact about minimal sufficient cause is that one can define *Structural Equations* that supply explicit unitary expressions for effects in terms of a selected subset of their causes. This leads naturally to a consideration of the difficulties in parametrizing *The Two-Factor Model*. I give an example with complete data in *Down Syndrome Example*.

Given a valid causal model, techniques widely used in biomedicine involve *Marginalization* and *Stratification*, and in these sections I argue against their use. An *Obesity Example* illustrates the issues.

I think one of the key areas in causation has to do with *Attribution*, to what causes does one charge an effect? I try to back up this claim by showing how attribution relates to *Indirect Cause*, both in terms of the *Probabilities* and the underlying *Structures*.

Every causal diagram implies a probability diagram, and while causation is seldom reversible, probabilities frequently are; *Reversal* shows how. *Gestational Diabetes Example* gives a practical application, and *More Reversal* summarizes the general situation of fallible

4

measurements and how they affect causal analysis. *Double Reversal* provides the argument and method for transforming retrospective studies into prospective results. *More Indirect Cause* gives some slightly more complex computations, and initiates the methodology for computing in general causal diagrams.

Dual Causation happens when a cause causes an effect and the absence of the cause causes the absence of the effect. Classical methodology has not discovered this distinction, but the minimal sufficient cause approach provides information about the impact on *Probabilities* and on the underlying *Structures*. Here it is argued that the odds ratio confounds harmful and preventive effects. Another neglected area is *Paradoxical Causation*, in which both the cause and its absence cause the effect.

It could be argued that one of the main reasons for having a theory of causation is to be able to justify experimental *Interventions*, and I examine how this looks from the perspective of minimal sufficient cause, and in particular what problems arise from counterfactual theories of causation. In *Causal Covariance* I introduce a measure that corresponds to the covariance in linear analysis, but which performs a similar function in the unitary algebra of causation. The general issue of time is not handled here, but I cannot resist at least indicating how *Unitary Rates* can be used to define times at which causal equations become satisfied.

When some variables are functions of others it is natural to imagine that the relationship is causal, but in *Functional Causation* I show that such a definition is problematic, and in particular that the prevailing notion of causation in the artificial intelligence community relies on some very strong assumptions. The *Causation Operator* maps any factor into its largest sufficient cause, and under some natural conditions on the notion of causation, this operator has many of the properties of a conditional expectation. In *Causal Modeling* a number of threads are tied together. I discuss the two probability models that one might want to employ, how to do likelihood inference for them (in both the prospective and retrospective design), and I give an example of a causal diagram using these models.

In *Dependence* I show how this illusive concept can be defined using the principles of minimal sufficient cause, and that together with the idea

5

of a natural imperative to solve causal dependencies, it can be used to construct a causal theory that obviates many of the problems raised earlier in the book. Finally, in *DAG Theory* I relate minimal sufficient cause to modern ideas of causation based on directed acyclic graphs.

In the *Epilogue* I deplore the sad condition of causal thinking and analysis in modern biomedicine, and then I point to some *Further Reading*.

Although there are not very many examples in this book, they are all from biomedicine and epidemiology, where I do my work. My intent has been to orient the narrative toward these fields, because they are perhaps in the greatest need of incorporating causal analysis into their daily work, and causal conceptualization into thinking about their disciplines. It is my conviction that we can make greater strides, and cover more territory, in pushing back the effects of disease and debilitating conditions, if we set as our goal the object of understanding how factors act in concert to produce effects. This path is fraught with complexity, but we are at least beginning to understand some parts of it. One approach to the path is the story of causation that unfolds on the following pages.

What Is Causation?

Cause is both a commonplace of ordinary life, and a mystery of the universe. On the one hand, we behave every day as though we were absolutely convinced of the existence of causal laws – rules that make things work in ways that we can understand and manipulate. On the other hand, it is an exceedingly difficult task to come up with a definition of causation that will satisfy everybody. The tension between the immediacy of our common sense idea of causation and the remoteness of a good abstract definition is one of the reasons that causation is so endlessly fascinating.

Some of the evidence for this division comes from fairly mundane experience. Those of us who read works on causation, and buy books or acquire articles on causal topics, are constantly amused at the number of times that the word *casual* is substituted for *causal*. We can laugh at phrases such as "the overwhelming importance of casual thinking in medical science", even as we know that the author is wincing at the way his or her words were turned. Perhaps there is an underlying cultural truth here, that in the current era most people have a casual attitude towards causal issues, which allows the slip to occur so easily.

Consensus Causation. And this leads to the question, given all the historical debate about the meaning of cause, and its necessity in our everyday lives, what is our consensus notion of cause? That is, among people who do not spend endless hours ruminating about ultimate meanings, but simply do science as part of their professional or intellectual lives, what do they mean by cause? If the Internet is any guide in this, then here is a definition that I found on a web site that seemed to claim some authority on the issue.

> **We believe that x caused y because, x happened, y happened later, and if x had not happened then y would not have happened.**

It is implicit here that x and y are events, so that events are somehow capable of causing other events. It also seems clear that part of the definition is that effects follow causes in time. Although these words seem meaningful, I think it can be argued that all of the rest of this definition is cloaked in obscurity.

To start off, why must we have that x and y both occurred? One way of looking at causation is to say that it involves rules, and at least some of those rules are of the form that if x happens then y will happen. This rule exists, however, independently of any of its manifestations. Even in cases where x has not happened, it seems sensible to say that the rule is causal, if it were the case that if x happened then y would happen. In other cases it seems possible to say that x has happened, but that y has not happened *yet*, because there is a delay between cause and effect. Why should this possible delay play no role in the definition? The distinction that is being drawn is between observing an instance of causation, as opposed to saying what the causal law is. The common sense definition given above confounds these two purposes.

And what are we to make of the clause that "if x had not happened, then y would not have happened"? This is one of those conditions that sounds eminently sensible, until one tries to figure out what it means, and then counterexamples spring up like daisies. Here is a story that illustrates what I mean:

> Person A is about to make a traverse across the Sahara in his Land Rover. The night before he leaves, B puts poison in A's water supply. Not knowing about B, C empties A's water supply onto the ground. The next day A sets off into the desert and dies. Who killed A?

To see whether B killed A, we ask if B had not poisoned the water, would A have died? The answer is "Yes, A would have died anyway" due to C's action. So B is not the culprit. To see whether C killed A, we ask if C had not emptied the water supply, would A have died. The answer is "Yes, A would have died anyway" due to B's action. So C is not the culprit, either.

This is not a subtle, tricky case. It is typical of the cases of putative causation that come up all the time. It shows that the common sense notion of scientific causation, according to many people, will simply not stand up to scrutiny.

Does Cause Matter? Do we need to be bothered by this? If our common sense idea of causation is logically unsatisfactory, does that make any difference? To answer this question I would consider another of the large philosophical issues, what is change? The student of philosophy will immediately be able to give examples of debates on the nature of change that go back to the ancient Greeks, but I want to skip over all of this to the mid 17th century, when Newton and Leibniz simultaneously invented the calculus as a method for describing change.

The fundamental methodological innovation of the calculus was to compute how far a particle moved during a time interval, divide by the length of the time interval, and then let the interval shrink to zero. When Newton and Leibniz introduced this idea, it was resisted by many. The notion that the ratio of things that individually vanish could approach something that did not vanish, or even something that made sense, was simply not within reach of most contemporary minds. Although the counter-arguments seem ludicrous today, at the time they carried some weight.

There is, however, an argument that can be brought against calculus even in the modern day. The computations rest on an assumption that time can be infinitely often divided into smaller and smaller intervals. This assumption is fundamental to the mathematics of differentiation, regardless of whether one differentiates with respect to time, or some other conceptually continuous quantity. What evidence is there, however, that time (or anything else) can be infinitely often subdivided? If this assumption fails, then does not calculus fail?

I think the answer is that in a practical sense, calculus does not fail, because the possible subdivisions of time (or of other things) are so far below the ordinary scale of things where we live, that for all practical purposes we can ignore the difference between very small (and measurable) time intervals and the limits that the calculus proposes. This is the answer given by history, in that the incorporation of calculus into engineering as a practical tool underlay much of the scientific and industrial revolution of the 19th century.

And so here we have an example of an enormously useful idea, unjustifiable at its philosophical base, that has played a huge role in the development of both engineering and mathematics. If there had been some particularly influential mind capable of making persuasive arguments against the Newton/Leibniz version of change before it had established itself, then how much of our subsequent progress in engineering and mathematics would have been lost?

Philosophers certainly spent no less time in the pre-Newtonian era thinking about cause than they did thinking about change. Perhaps there might have been a causal Newton, except that a mind did exist which challenged the fundamental notion that cause made any sense at all. This mind was David Hume, writing about a century after Newton.

Hume has, of course, been much read and interpreted. I can only give the impressions that I have from reading him, with apologies to those who have studied him professionally. Hume maintained that all of our knowledge arises from our senses. Anything that we can perceive or define in terms of touch, taste, smell, sight, hearing, or our kinesthetic sense, can be considered part of our knowledge of the external world. Anything else, that cannot be so defined, does not constitute part of our knowledge of the external world. So, when Hume considered causation, his first question was, what sense detects causation?

Readers of Hume have sometimes interpreted his stipulations of "constant conjunction" or "regular succession" as attempts to define cause. I think it is more likely that he posed these criteria as possible definitions for the explicit purpose of demolishing them. There is no sense (according to Hume) by which we can distinguish a regular succession that is part of a causal process from one that is not. Without such a sense, the idea of cause does not come from our knowledge of the external world. Having posed regular succession as the best attempt a rational person can propose for causation, Hume triumphs by showing that it is not cause by any of our senses. Consequently, for Hume cause is an invention of the mind, not grounded in experience.

In one of my fantasies, Hume would not have become obsessed with cause, but would instead have turned his skeptical eye on Newton's idea of change, and particularly instantaneous change. He would have ridiculed the idea of the infinite divisibility of time (or anything else), and cast out Newton's derivative as a function of mind alone, not related to experience. He would have succeeded in doing to change what he in fact did to cause. Change and its analysis would have been intellectually

10

suspect.   It would not have been a basis for engineering calculations, due to its philosophically shaky basis.   The industrial revolution would not have happened, at least not in the form that it did happen.

We have, therefore, many of the technological blessings and curses of modern life because there was a 17th century Newton, but no 18th century anti-Newton, and similarly, we do not have advantages of a good definition or idea of causation because there was an 18th century Hume but no 17th century anti-Hume.   Our lives are saturated with the occurrence of changes, to the extent that we do not even recognize this as being so, but we too often fail to understand the causal laws that make our world behave as it does.   So my answer to the question is "yes, cause does matter, and if hadn't been for Hume our causal technology might rival our change technology."

Causes Everywhere.   Writing about a century after Hume, John Stuart Mill expressed a completely different attitude toward cause, one which I think would have been shared by many scientists who lived both before and after him.   Unlike many other philosophers, Mill actually offered some canons for detecting when causation had happened.   I will deal with only two of them.

One he called the "method of difference", which amounts to the following.   Let x and y be two quantities, and let Z stand for "everything else", meaning all other quantities conceivably relevant to the discussion. If on two instances we observe that both x and y have changed, but all of Z has remained constant, then Mill concludes that either x is part of the cause of y, y is part of the cause of x, or there is some other causal connection that binds them together.   In order to shorten the prose, let us collapse these three conditions into one, saying just that "x and y are causally connected".   Another of Mill's canons is the "method of agreement", where in the two instances we observe that both x and y are the same, but everything in Z has changed.   Then again, Mill says that in this case x and y are causally connected.

Let us think how Mill's canons work in a very simple system, with variables x, y, z, w.   In the postulated two instances, both x and y change, and both z and w do not.   Mill's method of difference says that x and y are causally connected, and his method of agreement says that z and w are causally connected.   It seems to me that it is very difficult not to go from

11

this example to one in which we simply divide the variables that change in two instances from those that do not, and declare all in the first category to be causally connected and all in the second category to be similarly causally connected, although from two different canons.

Whether my extension of Mill's argument is correct or not, it seems reasonable to say that Mill regarded co-occurrences of change (or the absence of change) to be a signal of potential causation, and that the burden of proof was on those who wanted to say otherwise. His two canons were stated in such a way as to rule out the potential alternative explanations. Thus, if both x and y changed but nothing else (causally relevant) did, then what could be the explanation for their joint change except some fact of causation?

At the risk of extending Mill's argument beyond what he might have allowed, I would regard that many if not most scientists are Millsian in their hearts. If one persistently observes situations in which variables x and y move together in situations where other variables remain constant (are "controlled"), then what reason is there to say that nature has not decreed some law of causation that binds them together?

Descriptive Causation. Let us take a page from Newton and Leibniz, who figured out how to describe change, in the absence of physical or logical arguments for their invention of the *derivative*. Like them, let us figure out how to describe causation, even if we cannot justify by logical or physical arguments why our description is correct. In the same way that the axioms of calculus describe a conceptual world, which our actual world might approximate, let us try to find the axioms of causation and a theoretical causal world that our actual world might approximate.

From this "descriptive" point of view, the critical issue is, how should we fashion our tools of inference in order to uncover causes? The question shifts from "what is causation" to "how should we assess our observations in causal terms"? If we succeed at this enterprise, then we will at least be able to recognize that some ways of assessing observations do not correspond to any underlying notion of cause, and so we might feel free, in an extended Popperian sense, to disregard them. By refining our description of causation, and continuing to discard inferential strategies that do not uncover causes, we may get closer and closer to how the causal substructure of our universe might work.

Naïve Minimal Sufficient Cause

Before delving into the technical details, it is worthwhile to spend some time developing an intuitive idea of what minimal sufficient cause (MSC) means. There is no better way to do this than to study the work of two individuals who made fundamental contributions to the idea.

Mackie's Conditional Sufficiency. In both a 1965 journal article[1] and later in a 1974 book[2], John Mackie advanced a novel notion of cause. To set the background for this discussion, I will agree with Mackie that causation is a relationship that holds between events. One event is the effect, and the other is a cause. (Not *the* cause; *a* cause.) There are other ways of thinking about the setting in which causation is to be defined, and I do not want to be seen as suggesting that any of them are wrong. It is the case, however, that as causation is used in science, and in particular as it is used by individuals who nowadays think of themselves as doing research in causation *per se*, it is events that are seen as causing events.

In order to appreciate Mackie's definition, it is useful to know that historically a great deal had been made of the ideas of necessity and sufficiency as they relate to causation. Some would say that if C causes D, then every occurrence of C would be followed by an occurrence of D, which is just saying that C is *sufficient* for D. Others would say that for C to cause D, each occurrence of D would have to be preceded by an occurrence of C, which is just saying that C is *necessary* for D.

There is a convenient way to write these assertions. $C \Rightarrow D$ is used to denote "C is sufficient for D". A bit of thought shows that $D \Rightarrow C$ means that "C is necessary for D" (every time D occurs, if we look back we will find that C had to have occurred). The logical conundrum this leads to is that if C is both necessary and sufficient for D, then C and D are, in a certain sense, the same event. This is true because if we find out that either has occurred, we immediately know that the other either did occur, or will occur. The notation for this is $C \Leftrightarrow D$, which is read as "C is equivalent to D" (or, of course, "D is equivalent to C"), and means the same as "C $\Rightarrow$ D and D $\Rightarrow$ C".

Note that this logical difficulty plays fast and loose with our notion of time. Most people would be willing to grant that causes precede their effects in time. I am not going to make an issue of this, however, because time does not play a role in the constructive approach until a much later point in the development. Nevertheless, the necessity-sufficiency argument does lead to cause and effect being very tightly bound together, with perhaps only a time interval to separate them.

It is easy to see, however, that our ordinary commonsense notions of causation do not satisfy either the necessary or sufficient parts of this proposed definition. Consider the assertion "the cholera vibrio causes a fatal disease". I will argue that this is an example where the acknowledged cause is neither sufficient nor necessary for the effect.

First of all, it is helpful to patch up the assertion. One of the pitfalls in causal reasoning is to be led astray by characteristics of the language that is used to talk about causation, to get befuddled by what is said as opposed to what is meant. A more accurate rendition would be "exposure to the cholera vibrio causes illness followed by death". This differs from the more colloquial version in that it specifies two events, C = "exposure to the cholera vibrio" and D = "illness followed by death". We can differ about what exposure means, and we might even quibble about what death means, but I claim that the following argument holds for any reasonable interpretation of these terms.

To say that C $\Rightarrow$ D means that anyone who is exposed to the cholera vibrio will become ill and die. This is manifestly false, since throughout the history of our knowledge of cholera there have been many, many people who were undoubtedly exposed to the vibrio, but who did not become ill, or who did not die. In fact, one the Londoners who disbelieved John Snow's assertion that the water supply was causing the cholera epidemic in the mid 19th century intentionally ingested the vibrio-containing water with no reported ill effect. On the other hand, to say that C is necessary for D would require that all fatal illnesses were due to the cholera vibrio, ruling out the existence of any other possible causes of illness and death.

So here we have a clear-cut case in which everyone who understands and subscribes to the germ theory of disease believes in a causal assertion, but where the cause is neither necessary nor sufficient for the effect. It should be perfectly obvious that there are innumerable other examples that would make the same point.

Although Mackie didn't discuss cholera, we can imagine how he might have used that example to arrive at his definition of cause. First, he would have observed that there are many paths to fatal illness caused by other things, some of which might be microbial and some not. Let us use A to stand for the event that a person is exposed to one of these other (not cholera vibrio) causes of fatal illness. Next, he would need some explanation for why many of those who were exposed were unable to survive. He might have taken B to stand for the event that a person's immune system is too weak to throw off either the symptoms of infection, or to prevent death. No doubt there could be other reasons, but for the moment let us just rest with this one. Now Mackie would be in a position to assert

$$D \Leftrightarrow A \text{ or } (B \text{ and } C)$$

This says that illness followed by death is equivalent to either exposure to some non-cholera cause (A), or to exposure to the cholera vibrio and the lack of an effective immune response (B and C). Mackie took the above equivalence to mean that C is a cause of D. This definition completely eliminates the necessity-sufficiency bugaboo.

To generalize, Mackie would say that some C is a cause of some D just in those cases where there were two other events, A and B, so that the logical equivalence "$D \Leftrightarrow A$ or (B and C)" held. A consequence of this definition is that in those circumstances where A did not occur but B did occur, C would be equivalent to D. This is a kind of conditional equivalence, which generalizes our ordinary idea of equivalence.

Mackie went on to impose two additional conditions: that C is not a sufficient cause of D, and that B is not a sufficient cause of D. This led him to call his condition INUS, meaning that C is an Insufficient but Necessary part of an Unnecessary but Sufficient cause. Decoding this, C by itself is not sufficient, but it is part of "B and C", further "B and C" is

15

not by itself a necessary cause, but it is sufficient, and C is a necessary part of it.

It is this last phrase that is the most important: C is a necessary part of "B and C". This follows because B by itself is not a sufficient cause, so if C were deleted from "B and C" we do not have a sufficient cause. C is necessary for "B and C" to be a sufficient cause. Note that the use of the term "necessary" in the preceding sentence is not the same as "necessary cause," a fact that fogs up Mackie's condition quite considerably. Many of those who have misinterpreted Mackie have tripped over this linguistic twist.

The other condition (that C not be a sufficient cause) does not seem to play any role in Mackie's development of ideas, and indeed in his 1965 article he backed away from it within pages of introducing the INUS concept. He also immediately renounced the condition that "B and C" not be a necessary cause, thus allowing this as a possibility. These gyrations leave me with the feeling that INUS is a poor characterization of what Mackie actually wanted to say, and that the two actually important conditions are

$$D \Leftrightarrow A \text{ or } (B \text{ and } C)$$

$$\text{not}(B \Rightarrow D)$$

To be fair to Mackie, he did not make the strong assertion that these conditions *define* our notion of causation, only that they represent a part of what we mean by cause. I take his intent to be that any sensible notion of causation would need to include the above structure somehow, although it might involve additional conditions as well.

There is another way in which Mackie's conditions deviate slightly from what I have described. He was, along with many other philosophers, interested in accounting for causal occurrence in specific circumstances, so-called *singular causation*. That is, he wanted to be able to say "Mr. Fredricks was exposed to the cholera vibrio two months ago and this caused his illness and death" as a specific instance of causation. In this case he also wanted to say that Mr. Fredricks was not infected by any other micro-organism, nor did he suffer from any other cause of fatal illnesses, so that it was the cholera vibrio alone that was the cause.

Indeed, Mackie requires in a singular case that A not occur, but that both B and C occur in order for C to have caused D in that instance. I view this as a mis-step in the definition. The issue here is one of *causal attribution* - to what causes can the effect be attributed, and I maintain that this question has nothing to do with the definition of cause itself. This is, however, not the place to start that argument.

Rothman's Minimal Sufficient Causes. If Mackie's contribution was to distill and clarify the murky arguments of his predecessors into a workable theory, Kenneth Rothman in his 1976 article[3] presented a readable and practical application. As an epidemiologist, Rothman was interested in providing a framework for thinking about synergism and antagonism among causes of disease. To this end he imagined a disease event D, and a host of factors A,B,C,... that might play causal roles. He first generated conjunctions of events, such as AB (meaning "A and B"), and ABC (meaning "A and B and C"), and so on. In the disease metaphor, some of these conjunctions were imagined to be sufficient, in the sense that in any case where all the components were present, the disease would inevitably follow. Ignoring the problem with the indeterminacy of time in this account, we could write ABC $\Rightarrow$ D to summarize the situation, and we would then call the conjunction ABC a sufficient cause of D.

Rothman further imagined that every disease had a cause, so that if we were to list all sufficient causes, then their disjunction would be equivalent to the disease. To take a simple example (but only slightly simpler than the one Rothman used), we could write perhaps

$$D \Leftrightarrow ABC \text{ or } ACE \text{ or } BEF$$

This would give us three *causal pathways* to disease, represented by the three conjunctions.

We would now want to call each of the parts of the conjuncts parts of the cause, so that A, B, and C would be parts of the first causal pathway shown above. But there is a problem here. What about the case in which AB $\Leftrightarrow$ ABC? That is, if AB $\Rightarrow$ C, then the statement that AB occurred is exactly the same as saying that ABC occurred; the addition of the C term has a notational effect (AB is not the same set of symbols as ABC), but no actual effect in terms of the underlying events.

17

To be clear, suppose that G is some additional event that has nothing to do with D. Let G* be the complement of G (that is, the event consisting of all non-occurrences of G). Then we can write

$$D \Leftrightarrow ABCG \text{ or } ABCG^* \text{ or } ACE \text{ or } BEF$$

as another, equivalent way of writing the postulated representation of causal pathways. Now the irrelevant G has been catapulted to the status of a cause. One might leap to the solution, that this cannot be allowed because we have both G and G* as causes. This is simplistic, however, and I will argue that it is not only possible for G and G* to be causes of D, but that we are surrounded by practical examples where this happens.

Rothman's solution is much cleverer. Among the sufficient causes (or causal pathways) he distinguishes those that are *minimal*, in the sense that if we delete any of the terms making up the conjunction, what is left is not sufficient. This rules out the inappropriate G, since when we delete G from ABCG we are left with ABC, which is sufficient by assumption. Thus G is not a necessary part of the ABCG pathway, and so it should be deleted. That is, from Rothman's point of view we should only be concerned about *minimal sufficient causal pathways*, and the terms that compose them. He would, therefore, be willing to say that a factor was a cause of the disease if it were part of some minimal sufficient causal pathway.

At first blush it seems as though Rothman is saying essentially the same thing as Mackie did a decade earlier. There is, however, a very important distinction. When Mackie wrote "D ⇔ A or (B and C)" he did not place any further restrictions on A and B (aside from the one that B not be a sufficient cause). In other words, he did not tell us where A and B came from, nor how we were to construct them. In fact, he evidently considered it a strength of his approach that A and B could remain ambiguous. In Rothman's approach, to the contrary, we can see exactly where they come from.

Suppose, for example, we are interested in focusing on A as a cause of D in Rothman's equation. We simply re-write the equivalence as

$$D \Leftrightarrow BEF \text{ or } ((BC \text{ or } CE) \text{ and } A)$$

Now it is obvious that Rothman's BEF is Mackie's A, and Rothman's (BC or CE) is Mackie's B, when Rothman's A is Mackie's C. The critical

18

issue here is that in Rothman's system we can construct Mackie's A and B explicitly.

What is even more important, we can also focus on Rothman's B as a cause of D, or any other factor as a cause, and explicitly construct the corresponding Mackie equivalence. This means that with Rothman's approach we have a language for talking about *multi-factorial* causation, which (as we will see) unlocks the door to the solutions to a host of classical causal problems.

The Purpose of this Book. The remainder of this book consists of an attempt to take Mackie's fundamental definition of causal equivalence, and using the constructive method implicit in Rothman's approach, to show how any reasonable notion of causation can be extended and analyzed.

As a footnote to this section, one might ask why, if this seems like a worthwhile project, no one has tried it before. One answer is that both Mackie and Rothman were almost immediately attacked by critics, who left the rather strong impression that the systems they devised could not solve the problems they posed[4,5]. My feeling is that both critics erred, because they implied that because the methods did not work, they could not be fixed to work. Nonetheless, Mackie's INUS approach has played a diminished role in the subsequent literature on causation, and although Rothman's minimal sufficient cause concept is occasionally mentioned, I have yet to see any epidemiologic analysis of disease occurrence that used it.

References

1. Mackie JL. On causes and conditions. *American Philosophical Quarterly* 1965 October;2/4:245-255 & 261-264
2. Mackie JL. The Cement of the Universe: A Study of Causation. Oxford UK: Oxford University Press, 1974
3. Rothman K. Causes. *American Journal of Epidemiology* 1976;104:587-592
4. Kim J. Causes and events: Mackie on causation. *Journal of Philosophy* 1971;68:426-441
5. Koopman JS. Causal models and sources of interaction. *American Journal of Epidemiology* 1977;106:439-444

Events and Probabilities

Events and their probabilities play a very heavy role in modern ideas of causation. Several of the current theories of causation cannot even be stated without reference to probability. An approach such as minimal sufficient cause, which does not use probability directly in its definition, requires some kind of sampling situation in order to be useful for inference, and so again probability inevitably enters the scene.

Opportunities. As I indicated in the previous section, I view causation as a relationship between events. The first step down this path is to define the collection Ω of all *opportunities* for events to occur. A typical element of Ω is written ω. Ω and ω are the Greek capital and lower case omega, which we can identify with the word "opportunity". An *event* is nothing more than a subset of Ω. The elements of the set are the opportunities at which the event "happened", and those outside the set are those opportunities where it didn't.

There are several reasons for making this definition so formally. The first is Russell's paradox. If you do not specify Ω explicitly, then it seems as though you ought to be able to talk about sets like U = "the set of all sets that are not subsets of themselves". The problem is that if U is a subset of itself, then it does not satisfy its own condition for membership, and so is not a subset of itself. On the other hand, if it is not a subset of itself, then it does satisfy its membership condition, and so it is a subset of itself. If you specify Ω explicitly at the start of the argument, you cannot produce self-reference paradoxes such as this one.

A second reason, which is perhaps more pertinent to our goal, is that it is good practice at the beginning of a discussion of causation to say to what objects our causal statements apply. Philosophers who do not put themselves under this constraint frequently produce bizarre and irrelevant arguments, and especially quite ludicrous counter-examples to other peoples' definitions. Put differently, if we are allowed to switch Ω at will during an argument, then aside from the confusion we can create, we can also create some very bad reasoning.

Mackie himself was one of the few philosophers who imposed this kind of condition. He referred to Ω as the *causal field*, and he indicated several times that he thought this was the essential first step in a causal discussion. In subsequent sections I will widen his terminology to include some additional features.

Here are some examples. In a study of a disease, we might take Ω to be a well-defined collection of human beings, upon whom observations could be made. In this case, each ω could be one such person. If we wanted to take time into account, then we could take Ω to be elements like $\omega = (h,t)$, where h is the identifier of a human, and t is a time. Since an event is a subset, in this scheme an event would be something that could happen to various humans at different times. In a physics application we could take $\omega = (x,t)$ where x is a location in three-dimensional space, and t is again a time.

Although it is important to designate Ω, it is not necessary to put any additional structure on it for the purpose of discussing causation. In particular applications, Ω could be quite complex, consisting of elaborate combinations of simpler elements. For the moment, however, we simply assume that it is always defined.

Saying that event A happened at opportunity ω is denoted "$\omega \in A$". This latter is mathematics for saying that ω is an element of A. Saying that event A is a sub-event (or subset) of event B is written "$A \subseteq B$", which means the same as "for every $\omega \in \Omega$, $\omega \in A \Rightarrow \omega \in B$." Thus, the idea of a sub-event is essentially the same as implication. In the same way, "$A = B$" means the same as "$\omega \in A \Leftrightarrow \omega \in B$", so that set equality is the same as equivalence.

In philosophical discussions, events are often taken to be universals – that is, no specific Ω is assumed. This can be extremely risky, since even fundamental statements like "$A \subseteq B$" can be true for some choices of Ω and false for others. In a clinical trial, everyone told (A) to take treatment (B) might do so, because the investigators have admitted only compliant people to the trial, but in the wider community, telling someone to take treatment might not lead to them actually taking it.

The Boolean operators on events are defined as follows. A∪B is the *union* of A and B, and consists of all ω for which ω∈A or ω∈B. A∩B is the *intersection* of A and B, and consists of all ω for which ω∈A and ω∈B. I find the ∩-notation inconvenient, so in place of A∩B I will often write either AB. A* is the *complement* of A, and consists of all ω for which ω∈A is false. For formal reasons, the *empty event* is denoted ∅ and defined as Ω*.

The importance of the Boolean operators is that they allow us to make more complex events out of simpler ones. This is an example of a formal system, in that there are defined objects, and rules for combining them to obtain other objects. I will not go over the formal rules, since they are essentially the same as the rules of ordinary algebra, with which everyone is familiar. Thus, we can recognize A∪(B∩C) as the event that either A happened, or both B and C happened.

Statements that are always true in all Boolean algebras are sometimes extremely useful. Examples are:

$$A \cup \Omega = \Omega$$

$$A \cap \emptyset = \emptyset$$

$$A \cap \Omega = A$$

$$A \cup \emptyset = A$$

$A \cap (B \cup C) = (A \cap B) \cup (A \cap C)$	distributive
$A \cup (B \cap C) = (A \cup B) \cap (A \cup C)$	distributive
$(A \cup B)^* = A^* \cap B^*$	deMorgan
$(A \cap B)^* = A^* \cup B^*$	deMorgan

Further development of Boolean algebra can be found in texts on elementary applied mathematics, discrete mathematics, or introductory probability theory.

Because time ultimately plays a role in causation, let us look a little more in detail at cases where events involve time. Again using mathematical notation, [t,∞[conventionally designates the time interval starting at t and going out to infinity (that is to say, forever). Thus, stating [s,∞[⊆ [t,∞[is exactly the same as saying that s is later than t. Now let us think about pairs of the form (h,[t,∞[), where h designates a human and

23

[t,∞[a time interval. An event now consists of a collection of humans, each associated with a time interval. We could take D to be the event of death, so that (h,[t,∞[) ∈ D means that human h died (permanently) at time t. Similarly, B could stand for human-time birth pairs. This shows that this example can be used to describe temporal events that are permanent, or happen at most one time. More generally, we could have pairs of the form (h,T) where T is a time interval like [t,s[(or can be constructed from such intervals by Boolean operations). Then (h,T) ∈ A means that event A happened to human h during time period T.

Here is another example, which is more cosmological. We let Ω contain pairs (x,t) where x denotes a physical position in the universe, and t denotes time (on some fixed scale). Some interesting events are of the following form. They contain a given (x,t), and all space-time points (y,s) such that a physical impulse can start at x at time t and reach y at or before s. We can denote this event F(x,t). Assuming it is correct that no physical impulse can travel faster than the speed of light, and further that no physical impulse can travel backward in time, F(x,t) is the future cone of the space-time point (x,t). The event F(x,t) is all space-time points that causal processes arising at (x,t) can affect, and so we could call it the potential future of (x,t). Likewise, we can define P(x,t) to be all pairs (y,s) such that (x,t) ∈ F(y,s). This is the past cone of (x,t), or (x,t)'s potential past. There is a duality in these definitions, in that

$$F(x,t) = \{(y,s): (x,t) \in P(y,s)\}$$

$$P(x,t) = \{(y,s): (x,t) \in F(y,s)\}$$

Now F(x,t)∩F(y,t) consists of the potential future of x and y at time t, that is space-time points that could be affected by processes starting at both x and at y at time t. On the other hand F(x,t)∪F(y,t) consists of the potential futures of x or y at time t, all space-time points that might be affected by a process starting at x at time t, or at y at time t.

Speaking generally now, one usually assumes that the collection of events under discussion forms an *event algebra*, in the sense that any time we define a new event using a finite number of Boolean operations on events in the algebra, we get another event in the algebra. If we allow countably infinite sequences of Boolean operations, the result is an *event σ-algebra*. For any collection of events in Ω, there is a unique smallest event σ-algebra that contains them, and they are said to generate that event σ-algebra.

Probability. Formally, a *probability* measure is a function defined on events, taking values in the unit interval [0,1], and satisfying two conditions:

1. $P[\Omega] = 1$

2. $P[\cup A_i] = \Sigma\, P[A_i]$ whenever $A_i \cap A_j = \emptyset$ for all $i \neq j$

The first condition essentially says that some event has to happen (equivalently, $P[\emptyset] = 0$; the probability of nothing happening is zero). The second condition says that for any sequence of pairwise disjoint events, the probability that at least one of them will happen is equal to the sum of their individual probabilities. In order to make the second condition operational, it is always assumed that P is defined on a σ-algebra of events.

This is the formal definition, but making practical use of it often requires considerable care. My point of view is that it will only make sense to talk about probabilities in cases where there is a well-defined experiment that could, at least conceptually, be repeated an indefinite number of times, where one repetition would not affect another. In this case, the probability of an event is the same as its long-run relative frequency, which could (at least conceptually) be estimated to any limit of accuracy by repetitions of the experiment.

Perhaps one of the most important definitions for causal analysis is that of *conditional probability*. The conditional probability of A given B is defined by

$$P[A|B] = P[AB]/P[B]$$

if $P[B] \neq 0$, and is undefined otherwise. Whereas $P[A]$ represents the probability of A without knowing anything further, $P[A|B]$ is the probability of A after we know that B has occurred. This concept looms so large in causal theory that some researchers have tried to base the idea of causation itself on conditional probabilities.

Events A and B are said to be *independent* if and only if $P[AB] = P[A]P[B]$. When $P[B] \neq 0$ this is equivalent to $P[A|B] = P[A]$, meaning that being informed of the occurrence of B, we have no reason to modify the probability of A. Note that the definition of independence is symmetric in A and B.

Expectation. A *chance variable* is a function x defined on Ω, provided there is an event σ-algebra on the range of x such that whenever F is an event in that σ-algebra then $\{\omega: x(\omega) \in F\}$ is in the σ-algebra that P is defined on. The reason for this definition is that it allows us to talk about the *probability distribution* of x, which is nothing more that a list of all probabilities of the form

$$P[x \in F] = P[\{\omega: x(\omega) \in F\}]$$

When x is real-valued, we can define *integration* with respect to P. First, if x is the *indicator* of an event,

$$x(\omega) = \begin{cases} 1 & \text{if } \omega \in A \\ 0 & \text{if } \omega \notin A \end{cases}$$

then we define its integral by

$$\int x(\omega)P[d\omega] = \int x\, dP = P[A]$$

The second condition in the definition of a probability guarantees that if x can be written as a linear combination of a collection of mutually exclusive event indicators, then

$$x = \sum c_i x_i \Rightarrow \int x\, dP = \sum c_i \int x_i\, dP$$

The final step is that if a general x can be approximated by a sequence, each term of which is of the above form (linear combination of mutually exclusive indicators), then the limit of the integrals of the approximating functions actually exists, and so we can define it as the integral of the function x we started with. This requires proof, of course, and the reader is directed to a measure-theory oriented probability textbook.

In probability and statistics, the integral of x is usually denoted E[x], which is unfortunate, because it leaves out the information about P being the underlying probability. In cases where P does not change form from one assertion to the next, this is not a large problem. Note that the *expectation* operation E is linear

$$E[c_1 x_1 + c_2 x_2] = c_1 E[x_1] + c_2 E[x_2]$$

There are theorems that extend this linearity to series, but we will not need them here.

From our standpoint, a more interesting operator is the *conditional expectation*. Let x_1 and x_2 be two chance variables (defined on the same Ω). Under the sole assumption that $E[x_2]$ is well-defined and finite, it follows that there is a function g such that $E[x_2 f(x_1)] = E[g(x_1)f(x_1)]$ simultaneously for all functions f. The function g is essentially unique, and is denoted $E[x_2|x_1]$, the conditional expectation of x_2 given x_1. Remember that this quantity is always a function of x_1, the variable behind the bar.

The conditional expectation has several interesting properties, one of which is

$$E[c_1(x_1)x_2 + c_2(x_1)x_3|x_1] = c_1(x_1)E[x_2|x_1] + c_2(x_1)E[x_3|x_1]$$

That is, it has the same linearity property that E does, but now not just with respect to constants c_1 and c_2, but with respect to any functions $c_1(x_1)$ and $c_2(x_1)$ of x_1. This leads to the interpretation of $E[x_2|x_1]$ as the conditional expectation of x_2 if we were to hold x_1 fixed.

There is an important further reason why this interpretation seems right. It can be shown that there exists an object denoted $P[dx_2|x_1]$ which has the property that it is a probability with respect to x_2 for each fixed value of x_1. It can further be interpreted as giving the probability distribution of x_2 given x_1, in the sense that it can be used to compute all possible $P[x_2 \in F|x_1]$. It can *then* be shown that

$$E[x_2|x_1] = \int x_2\, P[dx_2|x_1]$$

In other words, the conditional expectation of x_2 given x_1 can actually be obtained by integrating x_2 with respect to its conditional distribution, given x_1.

Standard presentations of probability at the pre-measure theory level take something like the above as the definition of the conditional expectation. The presentation I have given is intended to provide some idea of the more general setting in which these ideas can be developed. (There are some measure-theoretic difficulties with defining $P[dx_2|x_1]$ when x_2 is not real-valued, but we will not encounter them here.)

27

The fact that probability can be understood in both its elementary and advanced measure-theory forms creates a problem. If one just provides results in the simple version, people can complain that they are actually much more general. But if we present them in their more general form, they will go over the heads of those who do not have the measure-theoretic background. My solution is to use *probability template* notation. In this notation pr(x) stands for the probability distribution of x, however the reader chooses to interpret it. $pr(x_2|x_1)$ is the conditional distribution of x_2 given x_1, again interpreted at the appropriate level of generality. Likewise, $pr(x_1,x_2)$ designates the joint distribution of x_1 and x_2. Rules such as

$$pr(x_1,x_2) = pr(x_2|x_1)pr(x_1)$$

can, therefore, be interpreted on different levels, depending on the reader. This will allow me to state results in the template notation, and even though it is a little sloppy at times, it will be understood by all. The way to think about a probability template assertion is that it generates a correct result, regardless of the level of understanding of the reader.

As a small example, consider the question, do pr(y|x) and pr(x|y) determine the joint distribution of x and y? One path to the answer is to write directly from the definition

$$\frac{pr(y|x)}{pr(x|y)} = \frac{pr(y)}{pr(x)}$$

Now sum over y to obtain

$$\frac{1}{pr(x)} = \sum_y \frac{pr(y|x)}{pr(x|y)}$$

showing that we can obtain the x-marginal distribution. A similar argument gives us the y-marginal distribution. So the answer to the question is "yes", provided that the expressions denoted by pr (probabilities or densities) are strictly positive. In fact, repetition of this same technique can be used to show that for a set of variables $\{x_1,...,x_n\}$ the n conditional distributions $pr(x_i|\text{all } x_j, j \neq i)$ determine the joint distribution of all the x's (again assuming positivity).

In the template notation we can also write $pr(dx_2|x_1)$ in the context of integration. We can also indulge in abuses such as $pr(x_1=0,x_2=0)$, which can mean a probability if x_1 and x_2 are discrete, or it could mean their joint density evaluated at (0,0), or a mixture of the two. Thus, the template notation is an informal way of indicating probability statements that can always be made more precise with more work.

Association. Independent chance variables are as un-associated as is possible. But checking independence can be both practically and theoretically tedious. A simpler notion of association can be built up from the idea of *covariance*,

$$cov(x_1,x_2) = E[x_1x_2] - E[x_1]E[x_2]$$

One motivation for this definition is that if x_1 and x_2 were indicators of events A_1 and A_2, then

$$cov(x_1,x_2) = P[A_1 \cap A_2] - P[A_1]P[A_2]$$

so that $cov(x_1,x_2)=0$ is equivalent to independence. If the covariance of two chance variables is zero we say they are *uncorrelated*.

In general, independent chance variables are uncorrelated. The reverse is not the case, except in some special circumstances. If two variables are binary (assume only the values 0,1) then uncorrelated implies independent. The same is true if the two variables are jointly Normally distributed. The coincidence of the notions of uncorrelatedness and independence is convenient when it happens, but it happens rarely.

In order to make it easy to talk about these distinctions, some relatively standard notation has grown up. We assert $x \amalg y$ to mean that chance variables x and y (defined on the same set of opportunities) are independent. When x and y are real valued, then $x \perp y$ means that they are uncorrelated. I have claimed that $x \amalg y \Rightarrow x \perp y$ always.

Here is an interesting application of these ideas. For a given y and x write $e = y - E[y|x]$. Recall that by the (measure-theory) definition, for any function f we have $E[ef(x)] = 0$. Taking $f(x)=1$ shows $E[e]=0$. It then follows that $e \perp fctn(x)$. This is another template notation, which means that e is uncorrelated with any function of x. The reason these facts are of importance is this: imagine that someone wanted to say that x was a cause of y provided that $y = g(x)+e$ where $e \perp fctn(x)$ and g is not constant. This would be a vacuous definition, because any variables (x,y) that are not independent are linked in this way. We cannot go through life interpreting conditional expectation relationships as causal relationships.

Conditional Independence. For the purposes of studying theories of causation, conditional independence is more important than independence. For chance variables x, y, z (defined on the same Ω), we write $x \coprod y|z$ and say that x and y *are conditionally independent* given z, if and only if

$$pr(x,y|z) = pr(x|z)pr(y|z)$$

This is, of course, just the definition of independence, but applied to the conditional probability distribution $pr(\bullet|z)$ (the $\bullet$ notation means "stick in here whatever kind of thing is appropriate", and is another way of talking about functions). It follows immediately that conditional independence is essentially equivalent to either of $pr(y|x,z) = pr(y|z)$ or $pr(x|y,z) = pr(x|z)$

When x, y, and z are indicators of events X, Y, and Z, then we use the expression $X \coprod Y|Z$ to mean the same as $x \coprod y|z$. In greater generality, if X, Y, and Z were collections of events, then $X \coprod Y |Z$ means that every event in X is conditionally independent of every event in Y given any event in Z.

Attempts to use probability to define causation usually take $x \coprod y|z$ to mean that x cannot be a cause of y. Let us use $\sigma(x)$, $\sigma(y)$, and $\sigma(z)$ to denote the collections of events that can be defined in terms of x, y, and z, respectively. Then $x \coprod y|z \Rightarrow \sigma(x) \coprod \sigma(y)|z$, but it does not follow that $\sigma(x) \coprod \sigma(y)|\sigma(z)$. In other words, in order to remove the relationship between x and y by fixing z, you must fix z exactly and not just approximately. This leads, of course, to philosophical problems with how accurately one can measure a variable. It is annoyances like this that occasionally drive one to hope that the universe is fundamentally discrete.

It should be obvious that we can extend these ideas, in order to say, for example that $x_1 \coprod x_2, x_3, x_4 | x_5, x_6$, which would warrant (among other things) the statement

$$pr(x_1|x_2, x_3, x_4, x_5, x_6) = pr(x_1|x_5, x_6)$$

Although it has been longer than other sections, this one clearly does not exhaust its topic. I will introduce other probabilistic ideas in subsequent sections as the need arises.

Unitary Algebra

Once one commits to the proposition that events cause events, then it becomes especially important to have a way of talking mathematically about how events can relate to events. The appropriate way to do this is in unitary algebra, which is both similar to and also different from ordinary algebra.

Basic Unitary Algebra. To start off, a *unitary* number is one that is between 0 and 1 (inclusive), so that it is in the unit interval [0,1]. A *binary* number is one that is either 0 or 1. Likewise, a unitary variable is one that takes values in [0,1], and a binary variable is one that takes values in {0,1}.

Unitary algebra has three definitions:

$u^* = 1-u$

$uv = $ product of u and v

$u \vee v = u + v - uv$

It is easiest to see why these make sense if we think in terms of event indicators. Recall from Section 4 that each event A in Ω has an indicator, which is a binary variable that is 1 at every opportunity where A occurs, and zero otherwise. Conversely, any binary variable is an indicator, in particular the indicator of the event where it assumes the value 1. Now for indicators, if x_A is the indicator of A, then x_A^* is the indicator of A^*, so that $x_A^* = x_{A^*}$. Further, $x_A x_B = x_{A \cap B}$, and $x_A \vee x_B = x_{A \cup B}$. This shows that unitary algebra applied to binary variables is exactly the same thing as Boolean algebra applied to events. We can choose whichever language we prefer (events or binary variables), and for our purposes I prefer the latter.

The $\vee$ operation is new, and perhaps requires some additional discussion. First, it is *associative*, which means that when we apply it multiple times, the order in which we apply it is irrelevant. Thus, $u \vee (v \vee w) = (u \vee v) \vee w$, and more generally the placement of parentheses has no effect on the outcome of computations that only involve $\vee$. Secondly, it is *commutative*, u∨v = v∨u, and more generally the ordering of terms is irrelevant in computations that only involve ∨. Of course, 0 acts as the unit, since u∨0 = u for any u.

Just as there is a notion of subtraction (-) corresponding to our usual notion of addition, there is a notion of subtraction (\) corresponding to ∨. The definition is

$$u \setminus v = (u-v)/v^*$$

provided v≠1, and we take u\1 to be 0.   Note that u-v is defined in conventional algebra as just that value satisfying v+(u-v) = u. In unitary algebra, u\v is just that value satisfying v∨(u\v) = u. Anything that can be done with - can be done with \.

For example, just as we have the concept of negatives, -u, we have the concept of \u. The definition of -u is 0-u, and so we can take 0\u as the definition of \u. Therefore

$$\setminus u = -u/u^*$$

provided u≠1, and \1=0. We can use \ and ∨ exactly as we usually use - and +. For example, no one is confused by u+(-v) = u-v, and so there should be no confusion about u∨(\v) = u\v.

When both u and v are binary then we can write u\v = uv*, and this latter expression is a little easier to deal with. Nevertheless, I will prefer to use the \ notation because it applies equally to binary and to unitary numbers.

Before going on to other aspects of unitary algebra, let me explain why it is important. Start with the familiar

$$P[AB] = P[A|B]P[B]$$

which is often called the multiplication rule, although it is actually just a restatement of the definition of conditional probability. This rule connects intersection of events with multiplication of probabilities. The question is, what is the corresponding rule when the left side above is changed to P[A∪B]? For the solution, observe that A∪B = B∪B*A and the two events on the right are mutually exclusive. Thus

$$P[A\cup B] = P[B] + P[B^*A] = P[B] + P[B^*]P[A|B^*]$$

$$= P[B]\vee P[A|B^*].$$

This rule connects union of events with $\vee$ applied to probabilities. It is the actual addition rule of probability, although another equation is usually called by this name.

Recall that independence of A and B means the same as P[AB] = P[A]P[B]. But from the result of the preceding paragraph, we could just as easily make the independence condition P[A∪B] = P[A]∨P[B]. To pursue this duality, suppose that for any A and B, I define π by

$$P[AB] = P[A]P[B]\pi$$

Then π is a measure of the positive dependence between A and B. When $\pi>1$ then P[AB] > P[A]P[B], or equivalently P[A|B]>P[A]. This is what positive dependence means, that when one of the events has happened, the conditional probability of the other is increased. Further suppose I define $\vee$ by

$$P[A∪B] = P[A]\vee P[B]\vee v$$

Although it is not so obvious, v is a measure of negative dependence between A and B. Substituting for the left side above

$$P[B]\vee P[A|B^*] = P[A]\vee P[B]\vee v$$

and \-subtracting P[B] gives P[A|B*] = P[A]∨v, so that v>0 implies P[A|B*]>P[A], or equivalently P[A|B]<P[A]. This is what negative dependence means, that the occurrence of one event lowers the conditional probability of the other. A further way to see the role of v is to verify that

$$P[A^*B^*] = P[A^*]P[B^*]v^*$$

Another important general formula from probability theory is the so-called chain rule,

$$P[A_1A_2A_3...] = P[A_1]P[A_2|A_1]P[A_3|A_2A_1]...$$

which is obtained by simply using the multiplication rule over and over. The corresponding $\vee$-rule is

$$P[A_1∪A_2∪A_3...] = P[A_1]\vee P[A_2|A_1^*]\vee P[A_3|A_2^*A_1^*]...$$

which is obtained by similarly iterating the addition rule.

One of the more famous rules of logic also holds in unitary algebra: deMorgan's rule is

$$(u \lor v)^* = u^* v^*$$

true for all numbers. The corresponding rule for subtraction is less well known:

$$(u \backslash v)^* = u^*/v^*$$

The one thing that complicates unitary algebra is the failure of multiplication to distribute over $\lor$. In general, we have

$$w(u \lor v) = wu \lor wv - w^* wuv$$

This shows that the distributive law holds provided that w is binary, but otherwise it does not. Another version of the lack of distribution is

$$w(u \lor v) = wu \lor (w \backslash wu)v$$

Although this may seem a bit bizarre, it turns out that in causal models there is a very precise reason for this equation.

For binary u, v, w it is true that $\lor$ distributes over multiplication,

$$u \lor vw = (u \lor v)(u \lor w)$$

but in general in unitary algebra we only have

$$u \lor vw = (u \lor v)((u/u \lor v) \lor w)$$

Unitary Probability Models. An important reason for employing unitary algebra concerns the parametrization of probability models. For example, let y and x_1 be two factors. Then I can always write

$$E[y|x_1] = P[y=1|x_1] = \beta_{0.1} \lor \beta_1 x_1$$

To see this, I merely have to recognize that it is the same thing to say

$$P[y=1|x_1=0] = \beta_{0.1}$$

$$P[y=1|x_1=1] = \beta_{0.1} \lor \beta_1$$

and then

$$\beta_1 = P[y=|x_1=1] \backslash P[y=1|x_1=0]$$

This shows that as the parameters $\beta_{0.1}$ and β_1 run through all possible values (that is, those for which $\beta_{0.1}$ and $\beta_{0.1} \lor \beta_1$ lie between 0 and 1), the corresponding probabilities of y given x_1 run through all their possible values.

It is worth recognizing here that while $\beta_{0.1}$ must be between 0 and 1 (a unitary number), β_1 only needs to satisfy $1 \geq \beta_1 \geq \backslash\beta_{0.1}$. This shows that β_1 can be negative, but not too negative.

Here is a very important algebraic equation that you can check by substituting the definition:

$$uw^* + (u \vee v)w = u \vee vw$$

Applying this to our probability model gives

$$P[y=1] = \beta_{0.1} \vee \beta_1 P[x_1=1]$$

Another way of showing this is

$$E[y] = E[E[y|x_1]] = E[\beta_{0.1} \vee \beta_1 x_1] = E[\beta_{0.1} + \beta_{0.1}{}^* \beta_1 x_1]$$

$$= \beta_{0.1} + \beta_{0.1}{}^* \beta_1 E[x_1] = \beta_{0.1} \vee \beta_1 E[x_1]$$

We will use this formula and its generalizations, as well as this basic method of doing computations, quite considerably.

We can extend this modeling process to two conditioning variables as follows:

$$P[y=1|x_1,x_2] = \beta_{0.12} \vee \beta_{1.2}x_1 \vee \beta_{2.1}x_2 \vee \beta_{12}x_1x_2$$

Because we can solve for the parameters in terms of the probabilities,

$$\beta_{0.12} = P[y=1|x_1=0,x_2=0]$$

$$\beta_{1.2} = P[y=1|x_1=1,x_2=0] \backslash \beta_{0.12}$$

$$\beta_{2.1} = P[y=1|x_1=0,x_2=1] \backslash \beta_{0.12}$$

$$\beta_{12} = P[y=1|x_1=1,x_2=1] \backslash \beta_{1.2} \backslash \beta_{2.1} \backslash \beta_{0.12}$$

it follows that this unitary parametrization places no restrictions on the probability model. As in the single-x model, some of the β parameters might be negative.

From the two factor model we can immediately compute

$$E[y|x_1] = (\beta_{0.12} \vee \beta_{1.2}x_1) \vee (\beta_{2.1} \vee \beta_{12}x_1)E[x_2|x_1]$$

There must be parameters α_0 and α_1 for which $E[x_2|x_1] = \alpha_0 \vee \alpha_1 x_1$, and so

$$E[y|x_1] = (\beta_{0.12} \vee \beta_{1.2}x_1) \vee (\beta_{2.1} \vee \beta_{12}x_1)(\alpha_0 \vee \alpha_1 x_1) =$$

35

$$= (\beta_{0.12}\vee\beta_{2.1}\alpha_0)x_1* + (\beta_{0.12}\vee\beta_{1.2})\vee(\beta_{2.1}\vee\beta_{12})(\alpha_0\vee\alpha_1)x_1$$

It is surprisingly more challenging to compute $E[y]$ in a symmetric way involving x_1 and x_2. Let $\xi_i=E[x_i]$ and $\xi_{12}=E[x_1x_2]$. Because we can re-write

$$E[y|x_1,x_2] = \beta_{0.12}x_1*x_2* + (\beta_{0.12}\vee\beta_{1.2})x_1x_2*$$

$$+ (\beta_{0.12}\vee\beta_{2.1})x_1*x_2 +(\beta_{0.12}\vee\beta_{1.2}\vee\beta_{2.1}\vee\beta_{12})x_1x_2$$

we have

$$E[y] = \beta_{0.12}(1-\xi_1-\xi_2+\xi_{12}) + (\beta_{0.12}\vee\beta_{1.2})(\xi_1-\xi_{12}) +$$

$$+ (\beta_{0.12}\vee\beta_{2.1})(\xi_2-\xi_{12}) +(\beta_{0.12}\vee\beta_{1.2}\vee\beta_{2.1}\vee\beta_{12})\xi_{12}$$

The next step is to extract terms of the form $\xi_{12}-\xi_1\xi_2 = cov(x_1,x_2)$:

$$\beta_{0.12}(1-\xi_1-\xi_2+\xi_{12}) = \beta_{0.12}(\xi_1*\xi_2* + (\xi_{12}-\xi_1\xi_2))$$

$$(\beta_{0.12}\vee\beta_{1.2})(\xi_1-\xi_{12}) = (\beta_{0.12}\vee\beta_{1.2})(\xi_1\xi_2* - (\xi_{12}-\xi_1\xi_2))$$

$$(\beta_{0.12}\vee\beta_{2.1})(\xi_2-\xi_{12}) = (\beta_{0.12}\vee\beta_{2.1})(\xi_1*\xi_2 - (\xi_{12}-\xi_1\xi_2))$$

$$(\beta_{0.12}\vee\beta_{1.2}\vee\beta_{2.1}\vee\beta_{12})\xi_{12} = (\beta_{0.12}\vee\beta_{1.2}\vee\beta_{2.1}\vee\beta_{12})(\xi_1\xi_2 - (\xi_{12}-\xi_1\xi_2))$$

When we add the four terms on the right, the coefficient of $(\xi_{12}-\xi_1\xi_2)$ reduces to

$$\beta_{0.12}*(\beta_{1.2}*\beta_{2.1}*\beta_{12} - \beta_{1.2}\beta_{2.1})$$

Dealing now with only the remaining terms, use the mixture equation to find that the sum of the first two is

$$(\beta_{0.12}\vee\beta_{1.2}\xi_1)\xi_2*$$

Also by the mixture equation, the sum of the second two is

$$(\beta_{0.12}\vee\beta_{2.1}\vee(\beta_{1.2}\vee\beta_{12})\xi_1)\xi_2 = (\beta_{0.12}\vee\beta_{1.2}\xi_1\vee\beta_{2.1}\vee(\xi_1\backslash\beta_{1.2}\xi_1)\beta_{12})\xi_2$$

Applying the mixture equation to these latter two gives

$$\beta_{0.12}\vee\beta_{1.2}\xi_1\vee(\beta_{2.1}\vee(\xi_1\backslash\beta_{1.2}\xi_1)\beta_{12})\xi_2$$

Putting everything together

$$E[y] = \beta_{0.12}\vee\beta_{1.2}\xi_1\vee\beta_{2.1}\xi_2\vee$$

$$(\xi_1\backslash\beta_{1.2}\xi_1)(\xi_2\backslash\beta_{2.1}\xi_2)\beta_{12}\vee(\beta_{1.2}*\beta_{2.1}*\beta_{12} - \beta_{1.2}\beta_{2.1})cov(x_1,x_2)$$

The most general model of this type can be constructed as follows. Let $N = \{1,2,\ldots,n\}$ and let x_i for $i \in N$ be the factors of interest. For each subset $A \subseteq N$ let

$$x_A = \prod_{i \in A} x_i \qquad (x_\emptyset = 1)$$

and then define the model as

$$P[y=1|x_1,\ldots,x_n] = \vee\{\beta_A x_A : A \subseteq N\}$$

An assumption that the model is of this parametric form places no restrictions on the probabilities on the left.

Random Effect Models. Minimal sufficient causation leads to models of the following form:

$$y = b_{0.1} \vee b_1 x_1$$

Here, $b_{0.1}$ and b_1 are factors, and so they have the same status as do x_1 and y. In the preceding section the corresponding model was of the form

$$E[y|x_1] = \beta_{0.1} \vee \beta_1 x_1$$

and because the parameters $\beta_{0.1}$ and β_1 were conceptualized as constants, this is called a *fixed-effects model*. But when we move to $b_{0.1}$ and b_1, we refer to them as *random effects*.

Since $E[y|x_1]$ always satisfies the fixed-effects model, there must be some relationship between the random and fixed effects. While this is true in general, it can become complex. The simplest case is $b_{0.1} \amalg b_1 | x_1$, because then

$$E[y|x_1] = E[b_{0.1}+b_{0.1}*b_1 x_1|x_1] = E[b_{0.1}|x_1]+E[b_{0.1}*|x_1]E[b_1|x_1]x_1=$$

$$= E[b_{0.1}|x_1] \vee E[b_1|x_1]x_1$$

There must be constants α_0, α_1, δ_0, δ_1 for which

$$E[b_{0.1}|x_1] = \alpha_0 \vee \alpha_1 x_1$$

$$E[b_1|x_1] = \delta_0 \vee \delta_1 x_1$$

from which we get the fixed-effects model

$$E[y|x_1] = \alpha_0 \vee (\alpha_1 \vee \delta_0 \vee \delta_1)x_1$$

This result would, of course, become quite a bit simpler if in addition we had $b_{0.1}, b_1 \amalg x_1$, because then

$$E[y|x_1] = E[b_{0.1}] \vee E[b_1]x_1 = \alpha_0 \vee \delta_0 x_1$$

which is a more interpretable fixed-effects model.

The two-factor random effects model is

$$y = b_{0.12} \vee b_{1.2}x_1 \vee b_{2.1}x_2 \vee b_{12}x_1x_2$$

It should be evident that the relationships between the b's , and between the b's and x's will determine the probability model conditional on the x's. The above equation is an example of the type that is required for minimal sufficient causation, and so we are going to have to deal with these difficulties. Since it is most illuminating to handle these interrelationships in causal terms, I will postpone their discussion to later sections.

The most general random-effects model is of essentially the same form as the most general fixed-effects model. Let $N = \{1,2,\ldots,n\}$ and let x_i for $i \in N$ be the factors of interest. For each subset $A \subseteq N$ let

$$x_A = \prod_{i \in A} x_i \quad (x_\emptyset = 1)$$

and then define the model as

$$y = \vee \{b_A x_A : A \subseteq N\}$$

I will refer to a model stated in the above form as a *structural model*, because it shows how y is literally composed of its specific components. Correspondingly, I will call the fixed-effects model the *probability model*, since it only defines probabilities. As I have indicated, a great deal of the work of causal modeling involves delineating the relationships between the structural and corresponding probability model. Whereas a purely statistical approach to modeling would just impose assumptions (like those I did in the two-factor model above) in order to make the relationships simpler, we do not have this easy maneuver available to us in causal modeling, because there is little reason to imagine that nature is interested in making the job of inference easy for us.

Nontrivial Implication

This is a very easy notion of causation to deal with[1]. In fact, it is so simple that it seems as though it could not contribute to any really useful version of causation. We will see, however, that it is more powerful than it appears.

The Causal Field. In order to set the stage, I first need to elaborate on Mackie's idea of a causal field. Recall that Ω stands for the set of opportunities at which events might occur, and that this is what Mackie meant by a causal field. To this, I will add a specific collection of factors **F**. Recall that a factor is a function defined on Ω that assumes only the values 0 or 1, and that each factor corresponds to an event.

The idea behind **F** is that it represents all of the factors whose causal effects I currently would like to consider. It may well contain factors I cannot measure, either because I have no good way of measuring them, or because I don't actually know about their existence.

For example, consider a hypothetical study to try to determine the causes of breast cancer. Here is a list of factors I would like to measure:

x_1 = first-degree female relative had breast cancer

x_2 = used birth-control pills

x_3 = had late menses

x_4 = had late (or no) childbirth

x_5 = carries BRCA1 gene

x_6 = has high intake of dietary saturated fat

x_7 = age above 50

x_7^* = age at or below 50

x_8 = age above 60

x_9 = age above 70

x_{10} = was exposed to pesticide during puberty

x_{11} = thin (low body mass index)

x_{12} = has dense breasts

x_{13} = breast-fed at least one child

x_{14} = breast fed two or more children

x_{15} = has physically abusive partner

x_{16} = has history of cancer at other sites

This list could obviously go on. It is also clear that it is incomplete in the sense that there are other factors that I would like to measure, if only I knew about them. (Some of these factors would need to be refined, but remember that this is only an illustrative example.)

The first interesting thing to notice about **F** is that it need not be closed under complementation. In fact, x_7 is the only factor whose complement is also in **F**. There is no prohibition against complements, it is just important to note that closure under complementation is not required.

The second thing is that **F** does not contain the factor constantly zero (which is just written 0) nor the factor constantly one (just written 1). This is a restriction that I will always impose on **F**.

The collection of all factors that can be made of products of factors from **F** is denoted ΠF. We also include 0 and 1 in ΠF. Based on the discussion of naïve minimal sufficient causation, we know that products of factors make up potential causal pathways. Thus, we refer informally to elements of ΠF as pathways. Of course, it is always possible that a factor from the original **F** is a pathway.

In the breast cancer example there are $3(2^{14})-2$ elements in ΠF. There are 2^{14} that contain neither x_7 nor $x_7{}^*$ (including 0), and then $2^{14}-1$ with x_7 and another $2^{14}-1$ with $x_7{}^*$. The number of potential pathways grows rather rapidly with the number of elements in **F**.

Finally, we denote by ∨ΠF the collection of all factors that can be made up of elements from ΠF using ∨. Again drawing on our understanding of naïve minimal sufficient causation, we recognize this as the collection of all disjunctions of pathways.

Nontrivial Implication. All we have accomplished so far is a language for talking about the factors we are interested in, pathways that can be constructed from them, and disjunctions that can be made from the pathways. The idea of *nontrivial implication* (NI) now comes into the picture with the following definition; for any two factors f and g.

$$f \xrightarrow{\text{NI}} g \Leftrightarrow 0 \neq f \leq g$$

This definition says that f is an NI cause of g if and only if (1) f is not trivially 0, and (2) $f(\omega) = 1 \Rightarrow g(\omega) = 1$, or in other words, at every opportunity where the event corresponding to f happens, the event corresponding to g happens, too. Note that this notion of causation is defined for all events, regardless of whether they are in F, ΠF, or ∨ΠF. As a matter of notation, I will signify the denial of $f \xrightarrow{\text{NI}} g$ by $f \xnrightarrow{\text{NI}} g$.

Now suppose that y is a factor, which I want to think of as a possible effect of causes in F. Define

$$C[y|F] = \vee \{f \in \Pi F : f \xrightarrow{\text{NI}} y \}$$

This is the ∨-sum of all pathways that cause y in the NI sense. $C[y|F]$ is, of course, an element of ∨ΠF, and it seems legitimate to call it "the NI causes of y generated by F". We have the obvious

$$y \in \vee \Pi F \Leftrightarrow y = C[y|F]$$

We now turn to a specific $x_1 \in F$ and the question of what role it plays in causing y. Define F_1 to be F with x_1 removed. Of course, ΠF_1 and $\vee \Pi F_1$ are defined in the obvious way, starting from F_1 instead of F. Define the *residual cause* as

$$b_{0.1} = C[y|F_1] = \vee \{f \in \Pi F_1 : f \xrightarrow{\text{NI}} y \}$$

and the *co-cause* as

$$b_1 = \vee \{f \in \Pi F_1 : fx_1 \xrightarrow{\text{NI}} y, f \xnrightarrow{\text{NI}} y \}$$

Now $b_{0.1}$ and b_1 are new factors in $\vee \Pi F_1$. The interpretation of $b_{0.1}$ is fairly clear - it consists of the causes of y generated by F_1. The key point here is that the pathways that make up $b_{0.1}$ cannot make any explicit reference to x_1, because x_1 was removed from F to make F_1.

41

There is a subtle point here that is worth the digression. Suppose that $x_1 \in \vee \Pi F_1$. This means that we can represent x_1 exactly with a disjunction of pathways, none of which use x_1. In this case $C[y|F_1] = C[y|F]$. On the left side we have what we would like to interpret as the causes that do not involve x_1, and on the right we have the causes that can involve x_1. In this case, however, there is no distinction between the two. Consequently, we have to be careful to say that x_1 was not *referred to* in constructing $C[y|F_1]$, and not say that x_1 is not *involved*.

A second subtle point is that some readers will be tempted to abandon me here, since I seem to be permitting causation to include silly cases, like those in which $x_1 \in \vee \Pi F_1$. I ask to have my purpose recalled - to take a given notion of causation and make it better. I do not require that the given notion be intelligent or useful, and it could even be silly. All I'm claiming to do is improve it (which may not be very much if it starts out silly enough). Virtually every philosophical tract on causation that I have read presumes that there is one and only one real causation, and that it isn't silly, so it is necessary to festoon one's definitions with all sorts of conditions and caveats to make sure it cannot be made silly by the causal hyper-critics. Since this point has paralyzed the philosophical discussion of causation, I would be happy to avoid it here.

The meaning of the residual cause is, therefore, reasonably clear. It is all the causes of y that can be generated from F without reference to x_1. The co-cause is only slightly more complicated. First, it consists of potential pathways that do not refer to x_1. Secondly, each of those pathways must, together with x_1, constitute an NI causal pathway to y. Lastly, the original pathway cannot itself be an NI causal pathway to y. Thus it seems reasonable to call $b_1 x_1$ the causal pathways to y that involve x_1.

Note that it is essentially the minimal sufficient cause argument that makes this definition sensible. Just looking at the definition, we cannot remove x_1 from $b_1 x_1$ and still have an NI cause, reminiscent of part of Mackie's INUS condition. To make the connection with Mackie even clearer, we have

$$C[y|F] = b_{0.1} \vee b_1 x_1$$

To see this, first observe that it follows immediately from the definition that $C[y|F] \geq b_{0.1} \vee b_1 x_1$. For the reversed inequality, let f be any element of

ΠF with $f \xrightarrow{\text{NI}} y$. $C[y|F]$ is the $\vee$-sum of all such f. If f is in ΠF_1 then it is an NI cause of $b_{0.1}$ by definition, and so $f \leq b_{0.1}$.

Otherwise, $f = gx_1$ with g in ΠF_1. If $g \xrightarrow{\text{NI}} y$ then $g \leq b_{0.1}$ by the argument I just made, and otherwise g satisfies the definition of b_1, so that $f = gx_1 \leq b_1x_1$. This completes the proof.

This brings to full circle one set of ideas. If we start with a well-defined set of factors on a well-defined set of opportunities (that is, a causal field), and we adopt the NI version of causation, then we can explicitly construct the two elements that are required for Mackie's definition of a cause (NI version). The residual cause is intended to stand for all causes not involving the factor of interest, although in silly cases it may fail to do this. The co-cause consists of all of those factors which, together with the factor of interest, constitute minimal sufficient causes.

The fact that we have a causal structural equation is important, because it permits us to demonstrate things about causation. For example, if $x_1(\omega)=0$ then $C[y|F](\omega) = b_{0.1}(\omega)$, so that any cause of y must be attributable to $b_{0.1}$. If $x_1(\omega)=1$, however, then the situation is more complex. We have $C[y|F](\omega) = b_{0.1}(\omega)\vee b_1(\omega)$. Clearly $b_1(\omega)=1$ must happen for any causation to be attributed to x_1. But this is not sufficient. If $b_{0.1}(\omega)=0$ then we can attribute cause to x_1, but if $b_{0.1}(\omega)=1$ then attribution is ambiguous; it could be to either or both of $b_{0.1}$ and x_1.

Many philosophers would want to resolve the singular cause question unambiguously in these cases. They want to definitely be able to say that x_1 was a cause of y *in this instance* ω, or not. But it is easy to see that the NI causal equation may not give them this answer. It may leave them in the ambiguous case where $b_{0.1}$ and x_1 have equal claim to be part of the cause. It is, therefore, clear that any philosophical approach that tries to solve the singular cause problem before solving the "definition of cause" problem is going in the wrong direction, from the minimal sufficient cause viewpoint.

We might want to say that x_1 is a cause of y if and only if $b_1 \neq 0$. This happens if and only if $b_1x_1 \neq 0$. This simply means that there must be some instances ω for which it would be reasonable to say that x_1 was part of at least one of the causes of y. Note that by this definition we are making "is a cause of y" pertain to a factor in general (like x_1), and not to any particular instance of that factor (like $x_1(\omega)$). As we study it in the NI case, causation can only pertain to factors, and questions about singular cause only have meaning (and do not always have answers) insofar as they can be derived from the causal statements about factors.

Reference

1. Aickin M. A logical foundation for the minimal sufficient cause model. *Statistics & Probability Letters* 1998;39(3):271-281

Tiny Examples

Before pressing on with more abstractions, we pause awhile to consider some small causal fields, where it is apparent what is going on. These examples are not trivial, however, since they indicate some counterintuitive results even for NI causation.

Figure 1. The effect y for Example 1
Shaded squares indicate where y happened.

For Example 1, let the effect y be as shown in Figure 1. Here the 3x3 table plays the role of Ω. We could think of the actual set of opportunities either as the nine squares themselves, some underlying population subdivided into nine groups, or the uncountably infinite number of points on the page enclosed within the figure.

For the factors F we take the three rows r_1, r_2, and r_3, and the three columns c_1, c_2, and c_3. I suppose that $x_1 = r_3$, so we are focusing on the third row as a cause. Check that the only elements of ΠF_1 that are inside y are $r_1 c_1$ and $r_2 c_2$, so that $b_{0.1} = r_1 c_1 \vee r_2 c_2$. Next, check that both c_2 and c_3 satisfy the definition of b_1. For example, $c_2 x_1 \xrightarrow{\text{NI}} y$ but $c_2 \xnrightarrow{\text{NI}} y$. Thus $b_1 = c_2 \vee c_3$. The causal equation is

$$y = (r_1 c_1 \vee r_2 c_2) \vee (c_2 \vee c_3) x_1$$

Note that in this case their is no ambiguity of causal attribution. Every singular instance is caused either by $b_1 x_1$ or by $b_{0.1}$, for the simple reason that $b_{0.1} b_1 x_1 = 0$. Also note that $b_{0.1} b_1 \neq 0$, so this stronger condition is not necessary for clear causal attribution.

Example 2 is shown in Figure 2. Here, $F = \{x_1, x_2, x_3, c_1, c_2, c_3\}$, where the c's are the column indicators. Check by inspection that the residual cause is $c_1 x_2 \vee c_3 x_3$, and the co-cause is c_2. Thus, we have the causal equation

$$y = (c_1 x_2 \vee c_3 x_3) \vee c_2 x_1$$

This happens to be another case in which causal attribution is clear.

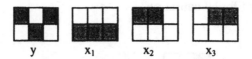

y x_1 x_2 x_3

Figure 2. Factors for Example 2.

In Example 3 we use the factors shown in Figure 3. Here we take $F = \{x_1, x_2, x_1^*, x_2^*\}$. The causal equation for x_1 as a cause of y is

$$y = x_2^* x_1^* \vee x_2 x_1$$

That is, the co-cause is x_2 and the residual cause is $x_2^* x_1^*$. What is remarkable about this example is that if we focused on x_1^* as a cause, then the above would still be the causal equation, but now with x_2^* as the co-cause and $x_2 x_1$ as the residual cause.

This illustrates the fact that it is possible for both x_1 and x_1^* to be causes of y. Although this seems paradoxical, it is, in fact to be expected. For a real-world example, the presence of water can cause death (under drowning circumstances, for instance), and the absence of water can cause death (by dehydration). The more one looks for cases in which, under radically different circumstances, both an event and its complement cause something, the more they seem to pop up.

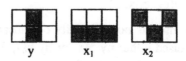

y x_1 x_2

Figure 3. Some of the factors for Example 3.

46

The next example is interesting for an entirely different reason. Again check by the definitions that the factors in Figure 4 give the causal equation

$$y = (x_4 x_5 \vee x_2 x_3) \vee (x_2 \vee x_3) x_1$$

The surprise is that $b_1 x_1 \xrightarrow{\text{NI}} b_{0.1}$. By our definition, x_1 is a cause of y, but its causal effect is completely masked by $b_{0.1}$. The consequence is that the above equation could have been written

$$y = x_4 x_5 \vee x_2 x_3$$

In what sense, then, is x_1 actually a cause of y?

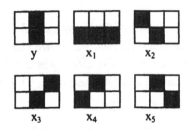

Figure 4. Factors for Example 4.

This example points up an extremely important distinction, the difference between a causal equation and a mathematical equation. The last two equations above are, indeed, identical mathematically. But the purpose of a causal equation is to show the components of a cause, even if some of them appear mathematically redundant. It would almost be better to define a "causal list" of component causes and not use the equation metaphor at all. While this would be more precise, it is messier, and not really necessary after we understand the difference between the two ideas. To answer the question, "is x_1 really a cause here?", I will peek ahead a little to say that the answer will turn out to be "yes", and the reason will be that x_1 is a purely indirect cause of y.

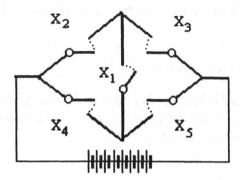

Figure 5. Electrical circuit for Example 5.

Example 5 leaves the world of little boxes and enters that of electric circuits. Figure 5 shows five switches, which we interpret as factors, with "1" meaning the switch is closed. The effect y is the flow of current in the circuit. As usual, we focus on x_1 as a cause of y. The causal equation is

$$y = (x_2x_3 \lor x_4x_5) \lor (x_3x_4 \lor x_2x_5)x_1$$

This example differs from the others in that $b_{0.1}b_1x_1 \neq 0$. For example, if $x_1x_2x_3x_4=1$, then the flow through x_2 and x_3 supports saying that $b_{0.1}$ caused y, but the simultaneous flow through x_4, x_1, and x_3 supports saying that b_1x_1 caused y. It is pointless to try to say that one or the other was *the* cause. My position is to say that causal attribution is ambiguous in this case.

The One-Factor Model

The Structural Equation. A causal equation is a structural equation, because it describes how factors combine to produce an effect. When we write

$$C[y|F] = b_{0.1} \lor b_1 x_1$$

we see how the residual cause and the co-cause together with x_1 literally produce at least some occurrences of y. When I said that we must start with the causal field (Ω and F), this was technically correct. In the tiny examples of Section 7, I always said explicitly what F was. The problem that arises is that if the F I select is too small, then $C[y|F]$ may only account for a very small proportion of y events. In other words, although the above causal equation is correct, it may not say anything about most occurrences of y.

There is a way to fix this. Again referring to the tiny examples of Section 7, I could always give expressions for $b_{0.1}$ and b_1, and so if I could observe every element of F then of course I could observe these, too. Suppose I were to imagine that, to the contrary, F contained factors that I could not measure. There are plenty of practical examples when this is the case, and in point of fact the case where all factors are observable is the highly unusual one. But once I allow unobservable factors into F, there doesn't seem to be any reason not to allow enough in to give a complete causal account of y. In other words, if some factors are unobservable, then saying $C[y|F] = y$ is actually an assertion that y is always caused by something that I might conceivably know about, and there doesn't seem to be any logical reason why I shouldn't do this.

An issue lurking here is that a causal equation may depend on what F one chooses. In fact, it is easy to give examples in which x_1 is a cause of y using factors F, but it is not a cause of y using factors G. To some, this feature of the minimal sufficient cause approach is unsettling, perhaps too disturbing to deal with. It is, however, an essential consequence of Mackie's reason for requiring a causal field in the first place. If we are allowed to vary which causal field we mean from one sentence to the next, then we can meaningfully assert contradictions. This means that our notion of causation is inconsistent. Inconsistent systems are very difficult to deal with, because a welter of mutually contradictory statements are all true. Failing to state a causal field (no less a definition of causation) is one of the favorite tools of the causal hyper-critics, since they then have the material at hand to counter any argument (even a valid one) with a counter-example.

The Probability Model. The upshot of this argument is that we might allow ourselves the convenience of writing the causal equation as

$$y = b_{0.1} \vee b_1 x_1 \qquad \text{causal}[\mathbf{F}]$$

at the expense of having $b_{0.1}$ and b_1 unobservable. By this maneuver we are in the position where we cannot compute these two factors. This does not mean, however, that we can say nothing about them. The additional tool we need is a random draw from Ω. If we can draw instances ω from Ω at random, then this implies a probability measure P over Ω. Under this probability measure, P[A] for event A means the probability that we draw an ω from A.

With P in hand, we can define parameers $\beta_{0.1}$, $\delta_{0.1}$, and β_1 as follows:

$$P[b_{0.1}=1|x_1] = \beta_{0.1} \vee \delta_{0.1} x_1$$

$$P[b_1=1|x_1=1, b_{0.1}=0] = \beta_1$$

The first equation says that the probability of the residual cause happening if $x_1=0$ is $\beta_{0.1}$, and if $x_1=1$ it is $\beta_{0.1} \vee \delta_{0.1}$. This involves no restrictions whatsoever. It is simply a way of defining parameters for this conditional probability distribution. The second equation focuses our attention on the probability that the co-cause happens, given that x_1 happened but the residual cause did not. I would argue that this parameter, β_1, is the measure of the causal force of x_1. It measures how probable y is under the conditions that the residual cause did not cause it, but x_1 happened and so was available to cause it, requiring only the additional occurrence of b_1.

We can put these two equations together as follows. First, if $x_1=0$ then $y=b_{0.1}$ and so we have

$$P[y=1|x_1=0] = P[b_{0.1}=1|x_1=0] = \beta_{0.1}$$

On the other hand, if $x_1=1$ then $y=b_{0.1}\vee b_1$ and we have to do a little more work. The key fact is that for any events A and B,

$$P[A\cup B|x_1=1] = P[B|x_1=1]\vee P[A|x_1=1,B^*]$$

Recall that I showed $P[A\cup B]=P[B]\vee P[A|B^*]$ for any probability measure P, and so it holds for the probability measure $P[\bullet|x_1=1]$, which is what the above equation says. So I can now write

$$P[y=1|x_1=1] = P[b_{0.1}\vee b_1=1|x_1=1] = P[b_{0.1}=1 \text{ or } b_1=1|x_1=1]$$

$$= P[b_{0.1}=1|x_1=1]\vee P[b_1=1|x_1=1,b_{0.1}=0] = \beta_{0.1}\vee\delta_{0.1}\vee\beta_1$$

What I have shown can be encapsulated into one equation:

$$P[y=1|x_1] = \beta_{0.1}\vee(\beta_1\vee\delta_{0.1})x_1$$

This is the probability model for the single-factor causal equation. It involves no assumptions beyond the causal equation and the existence of a random draw.

The IFR Condition. The difficulty with the probability model now becomes apparent. If I were to perform the experiment of making random draws, then I could accumulate any amount of precision in estimating two quantities,

$$P[y=1|x_1=0] \text{ and } P[y=1|x_1=1]$$

Without any additional conditions, this is all I could get from observations on x_1 and y. But this is the same as estimating

$$\beta_{0.1} \text{ and } \beta_{0.1}\vee\delta_{0.1}\vee\beta_1$$

It is evident just by counting that I cannot use these two pieces of evidence to obtain all three parameters. Unless I know more, I can't get any further.

The natural way to proceed here is to imagine that there is additional information, in that $\delta_{0.1}$ is known. If this were so, then

$$\beta_1 = P[y=1|x_1=1] \setminus P[y=1|x_1=0] \setminus \delta_{0.1}$$

and so I would have the causal force of x_1. Of course, in general there is no way to know $\delta_{0.1}$ without some additional assumptions or experimental evidence. The customary solution to this dilemma is to assume that $\delta_{0.1}=0$. This allows us to compute

$$\beta_1 = P[y=1|x_1=1] \setminus P[y=1|x_1=0]$$

Note that $\delta_{0.1}=0 \Leftrightarrow x_1 \amalg b_{0.1}$. Thus, the assumption necessary for everything to be rosy is that the factor we are interested in is independent of the residual cause. This is worth stating as a result:

$$x_1 \amalg b_{0.1} \Leftrightarrow P[y=1|x_1] = \beta_{0.1} \vee \beta_1 x_1 \quad [IFR]$$

This is a very desirable state of affairs, since the probability model is the mirror image of the structural causal model. One only needs to substitute $\beta_{0.1}$ for $b_{0.1}$ and β_1 for b_1. In order to have this, we must have IFR - *independence of the factor and the residual cause.*

Here is a good place to pause to consider one of the famous clichés of causation, "correlation does not imply causation". By "correlation" actually "association" is meant, and so the statement is that "$\beta_1 \vee \delta_{0.1} \neq 0$ does not imply causation". This is obviously true, because causation is equivalent to $\beta_1 \neq 0$, but consider the reversed statement, "causation does not imply correlation". Most people believe this to be false, but it is obviously true, since it amounts to saying "$\beta_1 \neq 0$ does not imply $\beta_1 \vee \delta_{0.1} \neq 0$". In general, causation and "correlation" are unrelated concepts.

Measures of Causal Force. The estimation procedure that follows from IFR is

$$\beta_1 = P[y=1|x_1=1] \setminus P[y=1|x_1=0]$$

This measure of effect (of x_1 on y) was put forward by Mindel Sheps in a series of papers[1,2,3] beginning in 1958. Her method was featured in one statistics text[4], but other than that it effectively disappeared from the biostatistical literature. She did not argue from causal principles, or at least not in the sense that I mean them here, but she showed some extremely interesting patterns that emerged if one used her measure rather than the simple difference between $P[y=1|x_1=1]$ and $P[y=1|x_1=0]$ or their ratio. The methods that eventually dominated in biostatistics and epidemiology were based on "odds" and "odds ratios", but as we will see, this choice may have been a mistake from the causal perspective.

Table 1 gives a concrete example. This issue here is the potential role of socio-economic status (SES) in causing women to undergo certain routine screening tests. Below the data are three effect measures. The first is $\beta_1 = P[b_1=1|x_1=1,b_{0.1}=0]$, the probability of a test given high SES and that other causes of having a test are not present. This is the causal effect of SES on having a test, assuming the IFR for this model.

The second measure is

$$\beta^*_{0.1}\beta_1 = P[b_1=1|x_1=1,b_{0.1}=0]P[b_{0.1}=0|x_1=1] = P[b_1=1,b_{0.1}=0|x_1=1]$$

This is just $P[y=1|x_1=1] - P[y=1|x_1=0]$, which most people take for granted as a valid effect measure. This latter measure takes the point of view that someone knows they are of high SES, and wants to know the probability they will have the test due to having high SES and not for any other reason, because all other reasons do not happen. In contrast, β_1 takes the view of someone who has high SES and does not have any other cause of a test, and asks for the probability that they will have the test (therefore entirely due to high SES). Both these measures have the same "numerator" (people whose test is caused by SES) but different denominators, depending on whether or not they might have any other cause. I will explain in a moment why I think β_1 is a superior causal measure.

Socio-economic Status		Routine Mammogram	Routine Cervical Smear	Routine Clinical Breast Exam
	Low	11/60 = .183	111/122 = .910	103/122 = .844
	High	35/90 = .389	121/129 = .938	116/129 = .899
β_1		.252	.311	.353
$\beta^*_{0.1}\beta_1$		.206	.028	.055
OR		2.84	1.50	1.65

American Journal of Public Health 1994;84:104-106

Table 1. Relationship between SES and having preventive tests.

The last measure is the odds ratio, defined by

$$OR = \frac{P\big[y = 1\big|x_1 = 1\big]P\big[y = 0\big|x_1 = 0\big]}{P\big[y = 1\big|x_1 = 0\big]P\big[y = 0\big|x_1 = 1\big]}$$

This is less defensible as a causal effect, for reasons that will be explained in Section 25.

Observe that for the first (causal) effect measure, SES has roughly similar effects on having a test, and if one were forced to say, then mammogram would be the test least affected, breast exam the most affected. Contrast this with the next row, showing the simple differences between the probabilities (since we can compute $\beta_{0.1} \vee \beta_1 - \beta_{0.1} = \beta_{0.1} * \beta_1$), in which the largest effect appears to be for mammogram and the smallest for cervical smear, and the difference between them to be quite large. Although the odds ratio is measured on a different scale, it gives essentially the same impression as the difference between probabilities.

The point here is that the causal measure β_1 suggests roughly similar effects of SES on having a test, regardless of which test is considered, and this remains true despite the fact that there are obvious differences in the probabilities of the tests. The other two effect measures do not distinguish between those who have and those who have not been deprived of other causes for having the test, and thus they make it seem that mammograms are virtually in a different category than the other tests. It was disparities such as these that first led Sheps to proposed using her effect measure, and we will both use it and generalize it below.

Although β_1 appears to give a more uniform effect measure in this special case, is there any reason to expect that it will do so generally? To answer this question, let us assume the IFR in $y = b_{0.1} \vee b_1 x_1$ so that $P[y=1|x_1] = \beta_{0.1} \vee \beta_1 x_1$. Now suppose that into this population a new sufficient cause a_0 of y is introduced, with $P[a_0 = 1] = \alpha_0$. We suppose that $a_0 \amalg (b_{0.1}, b_1, x_1)$, and we further assume that $a_0 \in \vee \Pi F_1$. After the introduction of this new factor, the causal equation is $y = (a_0 \vee b_{0.1}) \vee b_1 x_1$ and $P[y=1|x_1] = (\alpha_0 \vee \beta_{0.1}) \vee \beta_1 x_1$. It is obvious that β_1 remains the same under these conditions. In fact, all we really had to assume for this to happen is that $a_0 \amalg b_1 |x_1=1, b_{0.1}=0$.

With the difference measure, however, after the introduction of a_0 we have $P[y=1|x_1=1] - P[y=1|x_1=0] = \alpha_0 * \beta_{0.1} * \beta_1$, which is $\alpha_0 *$ times what the difference was before a_0 arrived on the scene. If we choose this as a measure of causation, then we have to live with the fact that the introduction of a new sufficient cause into the population, completely independent of all existing causes, changes the apparent causal effect of x_1. The more frequently the new factor appears in the population, the weaker the causal effect of x_1 will seem. In other words, even when we make all the assumptions that should leave causal effect unaffected, the difference measure shifts downward. We can see this in Table 1, where there might be additional factors causing women to undergo cervical smears and clinical breast exams, that do not cause them to have mammograms. This makes it appear that SES does not affect the use of the former tests to the extent that it does the latter test, creating a false notion that high SES somehow plays a stronger causal role for mammogram.

This same phenomenon plagues other measures of causal effect that have been promoted. For example, the "risk ratio" - in epidemiologic terminology - before the introduction of a_0 would be

$$\frac{P[y=1|x_1=1]}{P[y=1|x_1=0]} = 1 + \frac{\beta_{0.1}^*}{\beta_{0.1}}\beta_1$$

but afterward it would be

$$\frac{P[y=1|x_1=1]}{P[y=1|x_1=0]} = 1 + \left(\frac{\alpha_0}{\alpha_0 \vee \beta_{0.1}}\right)^* \frac{\beta_{0.1}^*}{\beta_{0.1}}\beta_1$$

Again, the pattern is that the more prevalent a_0 is, the lower the apparent causal effect of x_1, using this measure.

For the odds ratio, compute

$$OR - 1 = \frac{\beta_1}{\beta_1^*}\frac{1}{\beta_{0.1}}$$

It is clear that if we replace $\beta_{0.1}$ by $\alpha_0 \vee \beta_{0.1}$ then we will lower the OR. This is precisely what happened in Table 1, where the OR is lowered in the cases of the two more prevalent tests. In this example, a high OR was moved toward 1, but in other situations where the OR was already below 1, the introduction of a new causal factor would make x_1 seem like a more powerful (protective) cause.

The history of biomedical research is littered with examples in which different associations are found in different populations. One of the touchstones for causation that many scientists believe, is that if it exists, a causal effect should manifest itself to the same degree in different populations. What we have seen in this section is that if the MSC approach is right, then causal effects as measured by differences, ratios, or odds ratios, will indeed vary among populations that exhibit different frequencies of occurrence of causal factors completely irrelevant to the factor of interest and its co-cause, but that to the contrary, Sheps' measure will stay the same. If this line of argument is sound, then it suggests that at least some of the apparent confusion in the biomedical literature is iatrogenic.

The only way I know in which Shep's ideas have made any impression on epidemiology is through the *attributable risk among the exposed* defined as

$$\frac{P\big[y=1\big|x_1=1\big]-P\big[y=1\big|x_1=0\big]}{P\big[y=1\big|x_1=1\big]}$$

The argument in favor of this measure is entirely heuristic, that is, it depends on analogy rather than rigorous analysis. The numerator is supposed to be the amount of disease in the exposed population that would be left if the part that was caused by the same mechanism in the unexposed population were to be subtracted out, and then this is expressed as a fraction of the disease among the exposed. It can be re-expressed, however, as

$$P[y=0|x_1=0] \setminus P[y=0|x_1=1]$$

which reveals it as the causal effect of $x_1{}^*$ on y^*, under the appropriate IFR. In other words, the only measure, among those that epidemiologists have selected, which might have a causal interpretation as the force of x_1 in causing y, turns out to be a measure of the force of $x_1{}^*$ causing y^*.

This is a *preventive* measure, since it is the effect of the absence of the risk factor x_1 on the absence of the disease y.

A variant that is also used in epidemiology is the *population attributable risk*, defined as

$$\frac{P[y=1] - P[y=1|x_1=0]}{P[y=1]}$$

The argument for this measure is essentially the same as given above. Some algebra shows that it is in fact equal to

$$P[x_1=1|y=1]\frac{P[y=1|x_1=1] - P[y=1|x_1=0]}{P[y=1|x_1=1]}$$

This shows that the population attributable risk is proportional to the attributable risk among the exposed, by a factor that is rather difficult to interpret causally.

I have tried to make several important points in this section. The first is that a natural unitary probability model follows directly from the assumption of a binary causal structural equation. Secondly, the resulting model is correctly specified for the causal effect of x_1 provided that x_1 is independent of the causal residual, a condition that epidemiologists would call "lack of confounding". Finally I have suggested that none of the traditional epidemiologic measures corresponds to the causal model in a satisfactory way, and one can analyze their deficiencies in terms of the unitary probability model.

References

1. Sheps, M.C. Shall we count the living or the dead? *New England Journal of Medicine* 1958;259:1210-1214
2. Sheps, M.C. An examination of some methods of comparing several rates or proportions. *Biometrics* 1959;15:87-97
3. Sheps, M.C. Marriage and mortality. *American Journal of Public Health* 1961;51:547-555
4. Fleiss J. Statistical Methods for Rates and Proportions. New York NY: John Wiley & Sons, 1973.

Graphical Elements

The structural and probability equations of causation are important, but especially in complex systems it is extremely useful to be able to visualize the causal pathways.[1] In this section I want to introduce three graphical symbols, solid circle, open circle, and asterisk, that make it easy to translate equations into graphical diagrams.

Consider the first of the tiny examples of Section 7. The causal equation was

$$y = (r_1c_1 \vee r_2c_2) \vee (c_2 \vee c_3)x_1$$

Figure 1 converts this into a diagram.

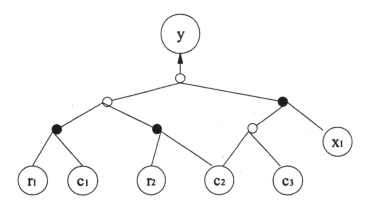

Figure 1. Conversion of Example 1, Section 7, to a diagram.

This diagram is the way computer scientists translate algebraic formulas into graphs. It is called a "tree", because if you turn the page upside-down it sort of looks like one. To see how the translation is done, first note that the structural equation can be viewed as the $\vee$-sum of two pieces, the residual cause and the part of the cause involving x_1. The open circle just below y represents this ∨-sum, and so it is read "or". Now going down the left branch we come to another "or", which is composed of two solid circles. Each of these represents a multiplication, and is read "and". So this branch "or's" two "and's", and each "and" connects two factors. The extreme left "and" connects r_1 and c_1, while the next one over connects r_2 and c_2. Now, going back to the top "or", just below y, the right branch leads to an "and" which connects x_1 with its co-cause. The co-cause itself consists of c_2 and c_3 connected by an "or". If this confuses you, just think about how you would compute the result of the structural equation. The parts you would compute first are at the bottom of Figure 1. These consist of two multiplications and one ∨-sum. Now replace the two solid and one open circle with the results of those computations, simplifying the tree. On the left, we ∨-add the two pieces and replace the open circle with the result, while on the right we multply two pieces and replace the solid circle. At the final step, we ∨-add the results of the left branch and right branch. Perhaps you can imagine why computer scientists like this representation.

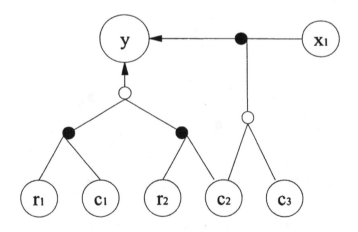

Figure 2. Although equivalent to Figure 1, here the role of co-cause and residual cause are emphasized.

But what works for computers often does not work for the human brain. The problem with Figure 1 is that while it correctly interprets the syntax of the structural equation, it misses the semantics. This is corrected to some extent in Figure 2. Here, I emphasize that there are two main causal pathways to y that I want to think about. One involves x_1, and it sticks out to the right of y, connecting to x_1 with a straight arrow. The co-cause now comes in from below and connects to the straight arrow between x_1 and y, showing its subordinate status. The other causal pathway consists of the residual cause. Graph-theoretically Figures 1 and 2 are identical. They differ only in emphasis.

The latter figure assumes, as I did in Section 7, that all the relevant factors are observable. In the graphical convention that I will use, observable factors appear in large circles (or sometimes other enclosed figures, such as roundy-edged boxes). One of the important ways that I intend to use causal equations permits some of the factors to be unobserved. If I imagine that r_1, c_1, r_2, c_2, and c_3 are all unobserved, then I would collapse Figure 2 down to Figure 3. Here, only the co-cause and residual cause are represented, and they are not enclosed because they are not observed. Figure 3 is, in a sense, the basic unit of causal graphics, because it displays effect, cause of interest, co-cause, and residual cause. In more complex diagrams it will remove a lot of clutter if I just leave $b_{0.1}$ and b_1 off the diagram altogether, the implicit idea being that they are there but not explicitly named.

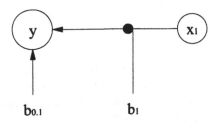

Figure 3. The fundamental graphical causal unit.

These examples show how we can use solid circle and open circle to represent a given causal equation. The asterisk plays the same graphical role that it does logically, to indicate complementation. While this is a great convenience, we have to use it carefully. Figure 4 shows a collection of causal assertions. They are paired, so the one on the left is the one we are thinking of, and the one on the right is how we graph it.

The important point in this figure is that there are no complemented factors on the right. The idea is that if the complement of a factor causes the effect (x* ⁻ᴺᴛ⁺ y) then we associate the asterisk not with x, but with the tail of the arrow that emanates from x. Likewise, if the factor causes the complement (x ⁻ᴺᴛ⁺ y*) then we associate the asterisk not with y, but with the head of the arrow that points to y. In some cases this won't work, and we must have both a factor and its complement in the same diagram just to keep things from getting too complex, but for the most part the asterisk convention lets us make much simpler diagrams.

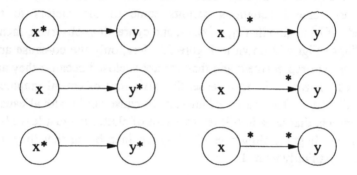

Figure 4. By associating asterisks with arrows, we can eliminate all complemented factors from a diagram.

As we go along, I will argue that effective use of graphs will build a bridge between how we think about the causal systems we want to study, and the causal analysis of those systems. We will eventually want to consider systems with multiple cause-effect relationships, and then graphs are not just decorative, they are essential. For now, I would like to show examples of how we might code some fairly simple causal systems into graphics. The object system will be a simple electrical circuit, using only switches, relays, a battery, and a lights.

In the simplest example, shown in Figure 5, y is the indicator of the light being on, and x_1 and x_2 are indicators of their switches being in the "on" position. The "on" position is shown by a filled box, and the "off" position by an open box. As shown, x_1 is on and x_2 is off. The elementary logic of the circuit says that y is on only when both x_1 and x_2 are on, or both off, since the parallel thick and thin lines at the right denote a battery.

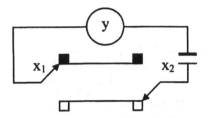

Figure 5. A simple electrical circuit.

The causal equation for this circuit is

$$y = x_1 x_2 \vee x_1^* x_2^*$$

and one version of the causal graph is therefore:

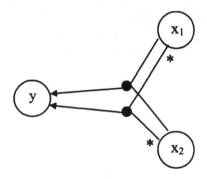

Figure 6. Causal diagram for Figure 5.

The top closed circle combines x_1 and x_2 with "and" to form one of the sufficient pathways, while the lower closed circle similarly connects x_1^* and x_2^* for the other sufficient pathway. Further co-causes and residual causes are not shown, because all three factors are measured, and implicitly $\mathbf{F} = \{x_1, x_1^*, x_2, x_2^*\}$.

Figure 7 shows a more complex example. In the upper part of the circuit, x_1 and x_2 must both be on for y to be on. In the lower part, if x_3 is

63

on and x_1 is off, then x_2 is forced on (the device just below x_2 is an electromagnet that is activated only when the lower circuit is closed).

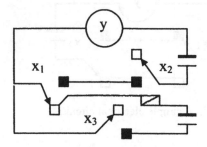

Figure 7. A circuit example with a relay.

Although you cannot tell it from the figure, x_1 and x_3 are *exogenous*, in the sense that they are controlled from outside the circuit as shown. x_2 is *endogenous* because it is (partly) determined by the other two switches. When x_2 is not so controlled, we imagine that it is caused by an exogenous variable $b_{2:0.13}$ which is not shown in the circuit. The causal equations are

$y = x_1 x_2$

$x_2 = x_3 x_1^* \vee b_{2:0.13}$

The causal diagram is

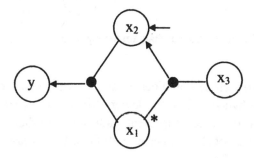

Figure 8. Causal diagram for Figure 7.

Note that the unmeasured, exogenous causal residual of x_2 is only indicated by an arrow, with the name of the corresponding factor left ambiguous. Also note that even though x_1 and x_1^* play causal roles, the asterisk notation allows me to show only x_1 in the diagram.

This example, simple though it is, demonstrates a number of interesting things about causation in general. For now, I would just like to point out one of them. According to the language we have been developing, we would say that x_3 is a cause of x_2, and we would also say that x_2 is a cause of y. Many causal theories then say that x_3 must be a cause of y, because causation is a transitive relationship. To be sure, they would distinguish x_3 as an *indirect cause* of y, while x_1 and x_2 are seen as being *direct causes*, but an indirect cause is not a cause of a different kind, it is a cause of the same kind with the single addition of an intermediate variable (x_2 in this case).

Let us then consider the following question. Is there any opportunity ω at which $x_3(\omega)$ causes $x_2(\omega)$ and then $x_2(\omega)$ goes on to cause $y(\omega)$? A moment's reflection shows that the answer must be "no", because we must have $x_1(\omega)=0$ for the first causal pathway to be activated, and $x_1(\omega)=1$ for the second causal pathway to be activated.

Considerations of singular causation suggest that x_3 is not a cause of y, but what does the minimal sufficient cause principle say? If we take $\mathbf{F}$ = $\{x_1, x_1^*, x_2, x_3, b_{2:0.13}\}$, then the only non-sufficient causes in $\Pi \mathbf{F}_3$ are x_1, x_1^*, x_2, $b_{2:0.13}$, $x_1^* x_2$, $x_1^* b_{2:0.13}$. It is easy to check that none of these together with x_3 is sufficient. Consequently, the co-cause of x_3 is 0, and so x_3 is not a cause, in the sense of minimal sufficient causation. This counter-example shows that minimal sufficient causation is not generally transitive.

Reference

1. Aickin, M. Graphics for the minimal sufficient cause model. *Quality & Quantity* 2001;35:49-60

Causations

Let us start by supposing that $\longrightarrow$ is a notion of causation. We will agree that there is an underlying causal field, Ω and F. We will also agree that $\longrightarrow$ is a *relation* between factors defined on that field and factors in a collection G This means that for some pairs (f,g) of factors with $f \in \Pi F$ and $g \in G$, the relationship holds, written $f \longrightarrow g$, and for others it does not, written $f \longmapsto g$. We will say that $\longrightarrow$ is *on* ΠF *to* G.

Sufficiency. In this section we will be concerned about properties which this causation relation might have. The most important of these is

Sufficient (S): $f \longrightarrow g \Rightarrow f \xrightarrow{\text{NI}} g$

This says that if f causes g, then first f is not identically zero, and secondly every occurrence of f implies an occurrence of g. In this case we call $\longrightarrow$ a *sufficient causation*, or an S causation.

The reason for making this definition is that sufficiency by itself cannot stand as a characterization of causation. Virtually everyone who has thought about it would require something in addition to mere "regular succession" – to use Hume's famous phrase – in order to have a truly meaningful notion of causation. Hume himself required something else, which he could not find in his own sensory repertoire.

An example that might help to clarify this is *mechanistic causation*. By this we mean that we have an interwoven collection of consistent rules that explain causes in some (but not all) cases, within the system we are talking about. For example, I might have a theory about the cells and other constituents that make up the human body, and according to this theory when a sufficiently great force impinges itself on a section of tissue, the cells rupture and the other elements that give the tissue structure are disturbed, nerve cells transmit electro-chemical messages to the brain signaling the occurrence, and physiological changes take place to restore the tissue to its former condition. In short, when somebody hits me in the arm, it hurts and eventually bruises. I have no difficulty identifying the blow as the cause of the damage, and I feel that I understand why because I believe the rules that I just outlined. For me, this was a causal occurrence because I understand and believe the mechanistic rules that explain what happened.

With this notion of causation, when I write $f \longrightarrow g$ I am asserting that there exists a string of mechanistic causes that form an unbroken chain between the occurrence of f and the occurrence of g. It might be the case that I can give an account of this mechanistic string, or that I believe in the near future that the missing rules will be found, and so a deeper theory than the one I have now will explain the string. In either case, an occurrence of f would imply an occurrence of g, and so I would have an S causation.

Cumulative. The next property that $\longrightarrow$ might have is

Cumulative (C): $f_\alpha \longrightarrow g$ for each α, and $\vee f_\alpha \in \Pi F \Rightarrow \vee f_\alpha \longrightarrow g$

The collection $\{f_\alpha\}$ need not be finite, and it could even be uncountably infinite. The use of the α subscript is intended to emphasize that there are no restrictions on the index set.

To elucidate what this means, let us turn again to mechanistic causation. Here, we would have a mechanistic string from each f_α to g. Now if $\vee f_\alpha$ happened, then one of the individual f_α would have happened, and so its mechanistic string would connect $\vee f_\alpha$ with g. But this just says that $\vee f_\alpha \longrightarrow g$. So mechanistic causation is an example of C causation.

It is, in fact, rather difficult to argue against C. If our notion of causation involves any kind of link to an effect that carries the connotation of "production", then certainly if each f_α produces g, then if any f_α occurs g will be produced. This is a rhetorical argument, and I cannot prove it in any sense.

Weak Transitivity. The next definition is often assumed rather casually:

Transitive (T): $f \longrightarrow g \longrightarrow h \Rightarrow f \longrightarrow h$

Said quickly, if f causes g and g causes h then f causes h. This sounds as though it should be true, but there are sensible notions of causation where it fails. Consider mechanistic causation. It is possible that the mechanistic strings only manifest themselves under certain conditions (Mackie's INUS again). It would be possible that all of the mechanistic strings emanating from f would arrive at g just at instances where no mechanistic string connected g with h. There would, of course, have to be some instances of g that were mechanistically connected to h, but they would not have to coincide with those from f to g. It might then be impossible to find any mechanistic string from f to h. My view is that transitivity is a very attractive mathematical property of causation, but I don't believe that it holds for most realistic notions of causation.

There is a condition somewhat weaker than transitivity that can be argued. This is

Weak Transitivity (W): $f \xrightarrow{\text{NI}} g \longrightarrow h \Rightarrow f \longrightarrow h$

In terms of mechanistic causation, this would say that once f happens, then g happens, and this connects to a mechanistic string producing h. In effect, the mechanistic string from g is connected to f by the fact that f implies g, and this induces the mechanistic causation from f to h. In my opinion this weaker form of transitivity is more realistic.

As I have informally indicated above, the properties C, S, and W will be used to denote characteristics of a causation. Thus, if I say that a causation is CW, this means that it is cumulative and weakly transitive.

Extension. Recall that the causation $\longrightarrow$ that I started out with is left-defined on ΠF. If $\longrightarrow$ is C, then we extend it to $\vee \Pi F$ by

$x \longrightarrow y \Leftrightarrow$ we can write $x = \vee f_\alpha$ with each $f_\alpha \longrightarrow y$

Note that $\longrightarrow$ must be C for this to work, since otherwise there might be a case in which $\vee f_\alpha \longmapsto y$ but by extension I change it to $\vee f_\alpha \longrightarrow y$. Thus every C causation, left-defined on ΠF, can be extended to be left defined on $\vee \Pi F$.

The extension only requires that there be *some* representation of x as a $\vee$-sum of causes of y. If $\longrightarrow$ is CW and $x \longrightarrow y$ by the above definition, then let $x = \vee f_\alpha$ as in the extension, and $x = \vee g_\beta$ for some other set of $g_\beta \in \Pi F$. We then have $g_\beta f_\alpha \xrightarrow{\text{NI}} f_\alpha \longrightarrow y \Rightarrow g_\beta f_\alpha \longrightarrow y \Rightarrow g_\beta \longrightarrow y$. The last step follows from the fact that the preceding step holds for any f_α, and so we only have to apply the extension principle by $\vee$-summing the f_α. This shows that

if $\longrightarrow$ is CW: $x \longrightarrow y \Leftrightarrow$ (if $x = \vee f_\alpha$ then each $f_\alpha \longrightarrow y$)

An important characteristic of extension is the following result:

if $\longrightarrow$ is C (CW, CSW) then its extension is C(CW, CSW)

To show this, first let each $x_\alpha \longrightarrow y$. Select $x_\alpha = \vee\{f_\beta : \beta \in B_\alpha\}$ with each $f_\beta \longrightarrow y$. Then $x_\alpha = \vee_\alpha \vee \{f_\beta : \beta \in B_\alpha\} \longrightarrow y$, proving C. Let $z \xrightarrow{NI} x \longrightarrow y$, with $x = \vee f_\alpha$, $z = \vee g_\beta$, and each $f_\alpha \longrightarrow y$. Then $g_\beta f_\alpha \xrightarrow{NI} f_\alpha \longrightarrow y \Rightarrow g_\beta f_\alpha \longrightarrow y \Rightarrow g_\beta \longrightarrow y$ because $g_\beta = g_\beta(\vee f_\alpha)$. Thus $z \longrightarrow y$, proving W. Finally, if $x \longrightarrow y$, $x = \vee f_\alpha$ with each $f_\alpha \longrightarrow y$, then each $f_\alpha \xrightarrow{NI} y$ and so $\vee f_\alpha \xrightarrow{NI} y$, proving S.

The story so far is that any C, CW, or CSW causation can be extended from ΠF to $\vee \Pi F$ while retaining its properties. As a result, we can always presume that any of the causations we are dealing with are left-defined on $\vee \Pi F$.

Nontrivial Implication (again). We now come to one of the key points in our study of causations. As before, we define

$$C[y|F] = \vee\{\, f \in \Pi F : f \longrightarrow y \,\}$$

Then we have

if $\longrightarrow$ is CW and $f \in \vee \Pi F$, then $(f \longrightarrow y \Leftrightarrow f \xrightarrow{NI} C[y|F])$

This statement is to hold for all $f \in \vee \Pi F$, but by C we only need to show it for $f \in \Pi F$. Then $f \longrightarrow y \Rightarrow f \xrightarrow{NI} C[y|F]$ by the definition of $C[y|F]$. Conversely, supposing $f \xrightarrow{NI} C[y|F]$ we have $C[y|F] \longrightarrow y$ by C, and so $f \longrightarrow y$ by W. This completes the demonstration.

From this result, it follows that every assertion about a CW causation can be translated into an equivalent result for NI causation. Since NI causation is simple, this means that all CW causations are actually simple.

Here is a somewhat stronger result:

if $\longrightarrow$ is CSW and $f \in \vee \Pi F$, then $(f \longrightarrow y \Leftrightarrow f \longrightarrow C[y|F])$

To show this, first note that it is easy to show SW $\Rightarrow$ T. Now if $f \longrightarrow C[y|F]$ then since $C[y|F] \longrightarrow y$ by C, we have $f \longrightarrow y$. Conversely, $f \longrightarrow y$ implies $f \xrightarrow{NI} C[y|F]$ by the preceding result, which is again by that result equivalent to $f \longrightarrow C[y|F]$.

MSC Causation. That is the end of the theorems, so it is worthwhile to consider what has been accomplished in this section. We start with a sufficient causation $\longrightarrow$ defined on pathways. Note that if we had a more elaborate causation that was not S, we could simply remove all pairs (f,g) for which f$\longrightarrow$g but f$\xrightarrow{\scriptscriptstyle NT}$g, and the remaining pairs in the causation relation would define an S causation. However obtained, I will denote this sufficient causation by $\xrightarrow{\scriptscriptstyle S}$. My fundamental assumption is that this would leave us with something; that is, the original causation had at least some cases of sufficient causation.

The next step would be to extend $\xrightarrow{\scriptscriptstyle S}$ to all disjunctions of pathways. The key assumption here is that $\xrightarrow{\scriptscriptstyle S}$ is cumulative and weakly transitive. First, the extension would retain these properties. Secondly, the extension would be equivalent to nontrivial implication, in the sense that the statements f$\xrightarrow{\scriptscriptstyle S}y, f\xrightarrow{\scriptscriptstyle S}$C[y|F], and f$\xrightarrow{\scriptscriptstyle NT}$C[y|F], are always equivalent to each other, where we remember C[y|F] = $\vee$ {f$\in$$\Pi$F : f$\xrightarrow{\scriptscriptstyle S}$y }. All of the results of NI causation are now available to us. In particular we have the representation

$$C[y|F] = b_{0.1} \vee b_1 x_1 \qquad\qquad \text{causal}[F]$$

where $b_{0.1}$ and b_1 are the residual and co-causes, defined in terms of our original causation $\xrightarrow{\scriptscriptstyle S}$. This is a considerable step forward, because now $\xrightarrow{\scriptscriptstyle S}$ has been extended to a non-sufficient causation (recall that x_1 is a cause of y if and only if $b_1 \neq 0$). There are now two possibilities. If $x_1 \longrightarrow y$ in the causation we started with, then we have recovered that fact, and established a structural causal equation. On the other hand, if $x_1 \longmapsto y$ then that causation did not satisfy the minimal sufficient cause principle, and so we have improved it so that it does.

Because of these results, I will assume in what follows that the causation $\longrightarrow$ in question is CW, generates an S causation, which I denote $\xrightarrow{\scriptscriptstyle S}$ and which is then automatically CSW, this is in turn extended as above, and has been brought into conformity with the minimal sufficient cause principle through its relationship with nontrivial implication. This gives me some new notation, which we have to be careful of. When I write "x $\longrightarrow$ y [F]" I mean the same thing as "C[y|F] = $b_{0.1} \vee b_1 x_1$ causal[F] ($b_1 \neq 0$)", which I could also write as "$b_{0.1} \vee b_1 x_1$ $\xrightarrow{\scriptscriptstyle S}$ y [F] ($b_1 \neq 0$)". It is important in this latter usage to keep in mind that the [F] notation indicates a causal equation, so it is implied that $b_{0.1}$ is the residual cause, and b_1 is the co-cause. Also remember that C[y|F] stands for the sufficient causes of y generated by F, C[y|F] = $\vee$ {f$\in$$\Pi$F : f$\xrightarrow{\scriptscriptstyle S}$y }.

When I prove things about this causation, I can use its relationship to NI, which is an easier causation to think about than the abstract CSW ideas. In order to bundle all of these ideas into a convenient phrase, I will simply say that " $\longrightarrow$ is MSC".

The preceding paragraph summarizes this section. It is important because it states an assumption that is in force throughout the remainder of the book.

Structural Equations

In Section 6 we saw how to develop a structural causal equation for a single factor, and in the preceding section we saw that for an MSC causation $\longrightarrow$ this could be written as $b_{0.1} \lor b_1 x_1 \dashrightarrow y$ [F], where the [F] notation indicates the presence of the co-cause and residual cause. In this section I want to do the same thing for a collection of factors $x_1,..,x_n$. In order to be of use, the x's would generally be observable, although that is not necessary.

The General Structural Equation. To make the pathway notation a little easier, let me write $N = \{1,...,n\}$ for the set of subscripts, and for each $A \subseteq N$ we will use x_A for the product of the corresponding x's, so

$$x_A = \Pi\{x_i : i \in A\}$$

with the convention that $x_\varnothing = 1$. I will also write F_A for F with $\{x_i : i \in A\}$ removed.

The residual cause with respect to this collection of x's is

$$b_0 = b_\varnothing = C[y|F_N] = \lor\{f \in \Pi F_N : f \dashrightarrow y\}$$

That is, b_0 consists of all sufficient causes of y that can be constructed without reference to any of the x's. A typical co-cause is defined by

$$b_A = \lor\{f \in \Pi F_N : f x_A \dashrightarrow y, f x_B \not\dashrightarrow y \text{ for all } B \subset A\}$$

Note here that $\subset$ denotes a strict subset, so that in the brackets B cannot be A. Every pathway in this definition is one for which x_A is a necessary (in Mackie's INUS sense) component, because deleting any x from x_A renders it not a cause, according to the second part of the condition.

The main consequence of these definitions is

$$C[y|F] = \lor b_A x_A \qquad \text{causal}[F]$$

The assertion here is the equation; the "causal[F]" part merely indicates how I am going to refer to this result. Here is the demonstration. First $C[y|F] \geq \lor b_A x_A$ immediately from the definition. For the reversed inequality, let $f \in \Pi F$ with $f \dashrightarrow y$. It suffices to show $f \leq \lor b_A x_A$, since

C[y|F] is the ∨-sum of such f. Now we must have $f = dx_D$ for some $D \subseteq N$ and $d \in \Pi F_N$. We know $dx_D \overset{s}{\dashrightarrow} y$, and so if $dx_B \overset{s}{\dashrightarrow} y$ for all $B \subset D$, then d is in the definition of b_D and we are done. Otherwise, select a $B \subset D$ for which $dx_B \overset{s}{\dashrightarrow} y$. We now iterate the above argument, at each step either finding that d is in the definition of a co-cause, or proceeding to a strictly smaller set of indices. This procedure either ends with d in the definition of some co-cause B, whence $dx_A \leq dx_B \leq b_B x_B$, or we get $d \overset{s}{\dashrightarrow} y$ so that d is in the definition of b_0. This finishes the demonstration.

An alternative way to write the causal equation is

$$\vee b_A x_A \overset{s}{\dashrightarrow} y \quad [F]$$

This brings another collection of ideas full circle. Recall that Rothman postulated that all of the causes of a disease could be broken into the minimal sufficient causes, and then he said that each component of a minimal sufficient cause was a cause. We have now proved that for MSC notions of cause, this decomposition is always true. Moreover, we have obtained a causal relationship that highlights the roles played by the factors (x's) that we are particularly interested in. We could also regard that the above causal relationship generalizes Mackie's condition for causation. These considerations suggest that it would now be legitimate to write

$$x_A \longrightarrow y \Leftrightarrow b_A \neq 0$$

We would read this as "x_A is a cause of y", although we might need to make reference to F, since changing F can change the causal relationship.

It is critical to see that only now for the first time do we have a constructive notion of causation that is not sufficient. In other words, the constructionist program is to start with a sufficient causation, and then through application of the minimal sufficient cause principle to extend it to a causation, which will usually not be sufficient. It may be of some interest to consider how one might characterize the causation that results, without any reference to how it was constructed. That is, how could we give a general definition of causation that is accurate, but does not recapitulate our construction? My feeling is that this is a very hard problem, which explains why there are so many different definitions of causation that fall short.

Notation for Small Cases. The notation that I used above was tailored for the general result on causal structural equations, but in actual cases another notation works better. We have already seen a little bit of it in $b_{0.1} \vee b_1 x_1 \dashrightarrow y$ [F]. In the case of $N=\{1,2\}$, the notation I would use is

$$b_{0.12} \vee b_{1.2} x_1 \vee b_{2.1} x_2 \vee b_{12} x_1 x_2 \dashrightarrow y \quad [F]$$

The subscripts appearing before the dot indicate which factors appear in the product, with 0 denoting the residual cause. The subscripts after the dot indicate the others that are in the causal relationship. Thus, I can always tell by looking at this compound subscript what the complete set of factors is. This notation is extremely convenient for distinguishing situations in which the factors of interest (x's) change, as we will see many times.

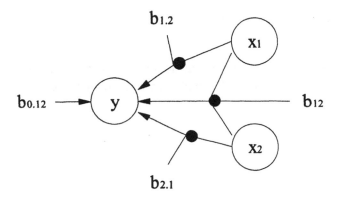

Figure 1. The general causal diagram for two factors.

The graphical representation of the causal relationship is shown in Figure 1. In keeping with my conventions, the b's do not appear enclosed, since they generally will not be observable, although this is not a requirement. In diagrams more complex than this, I would include the arrows associated with the b's, but not actually include the b's themselves, just as a device for reducing clutter. Recall that the solid circles stand for conjunction of all the elements that lead into them. Thus, the three arrows toward y from the right stand for the three major sets of causal pathways, those in which x_1 is necessary, those in which x_2 is necessary, and those in which both x_1 and x_2 are necessary. The single arrow from the left represents all other pathways, meaning those that do not refer to x_1 or x_2.

Disjunctive Forms. It is important to distinguish a structural causal equation from a so-called disjunctive form. Saying that $y \in \vee\Pi F$ is saying nothing more than that y can be represented as a disjunction ($\vee$-sum) of products of elements of **F**. There may be many such representations of a given y, and none of them need have any causal significance. For example, we might be able to write

$$y = x_1x_2 \vee x_3x_4 \vee x_5$$

in which x_1 is not the co-cause of x_2, and $x_3x_4 \vee x_5$ is not the residual cause with respect to x_2. In fact, it might be the case that $x_1x_2 \overset{s}{\nrightarrow} y$ but $x_3x_4 \overset{s}{\rightarrow} y$ and $x_5 \overset{s}{\rightarrow} y$ so that the causal equation is

$$x_3x_4 \vee x_5 \overset{s}{\rightarrow} y \quad [\mathbf{F}]$$

and the structural equation is

$$C[y|\mathbf{F}] = x_3x_4 \vee x_5$$

As always, the issue is that a given notion of sufficient causation may involve something in addition to simple nontrivial implication.

The Two-Factor Model

We start with the MSC causal relationship

$$b_{0.12} \vee b_{1.2}x_1 \vee b_{2.1}x_2 \vee b_{12}x_1x_2 \overset{\bullet}{\longrightarrow} y \quad [\mathbf{F}]$$

As I observed in Section 8, the notation will be a little easier (and there is no real philosophical difference) if I assume that $\mathbf{F}$ is sufficiently rich that $y \in \vee \Pi \mathbf{F}$. This allows me to write

$$y = b_{0.12} \vee b_{1.2}x_1 \vee b_{2.1}x_2 \vee b_{12}x_1x_2 \qquad \text{causal}[\mathbf{F}]$$

An equivalent maneuver would be to replace $C[y|\mathbf{F}]$ with the symbol "y" standing for "all causes of y in $\mathbf{F}$", again creating no confusion but simplifying notation.

The purpose of this section is to investigate the issues of parametrization of the probability model, using P to stand for a probability measure representing a random draw from the population of opportunities Ω. This task is somewhat more trying than it is for the one-factor model. The complete set of parameters is defined as follows:

$$P[b_{0.12}=1|x_1,x_2] = \beta_{0.12} \vee \delta_{0.1.2}x_1 \vee \delta_{0.2.1}x_2 \vee \delta_{0.12}x_1x_2$$

$$P[b_{1.2}=1|x_1=1,x_2,b_{0.12}=0] = \beta_{1.2} \vee \delta_{2.1}x_2$$

$$P[b_{2.1}=1|x_1,x_2=1,b_{0.12}=0] = \beta_{2.1} \vee \delta_{1.2}x_1$$

$$P[b_{1.2} \vee b_{2.1}=1|x_1=1,x_2=1,b_{0.12}=0] = \beta_{1.2} \vee \delta_{2.1} \vee \beta_{2.1} \vee \delta_{1.2} \vee \delta_{12}$$

$$P[b_{12}=1|x_1=1,x_2=1,b_{1.2}=0,b_{2.1}=0,b_{0.12}=0] = \beta_{12}$$

We will take some time to go through these, with the intent of finding their interpretations. But first of all, note that the probability distributions $P[y=1|x_1,x_2]$ require exactly four parameters. You will observe that there are four β's, and six δ's. As the numbers suggest, the β's are the parameters with causal interpretations, and the δ's are nuisances. Since the δ's will actually be present in real world situations, it is necessary to understand them, even if we would prefer that they weren't there.

The first equation permits relationships between the x's and the residual cause,

$$P[b_{0.12}=1|x_1,x_2] = \beta_{0.12} \vee \delta_{0.1.2}x_1 \vee \delta_{0.2.1}x_2 \vee \delta_{0.12}x_1x_2$$

Note the elaborate double-dot subscript notation on the δ's, making them notationally as well as inferentially unattractive. Setting all of the δ's equal to zero here is IFR - *independence of factors and residuals* condition, and it is equivalent to the independence assertion

$$b_{0.12} \perp\!\!\!\perp (x_1,x_2) \quad \text{IFR}$$

The next pair of equations

$$P[b_{1.2}=1|x_1=1,x_2,b_{0.12}=0] = \beta_{1.2} \vee \delta_{2.1}x_2$$

$$P[b_{2.1}=1|x_1,x_2=1,b_{0.12}=0] = \beta_{2.1} \vee \delta_{1.2}x_1$$

are very similar to the definition of β_1 and β_2, with the complication that there is another factor that may play a role. Thus, in the first equation we must take into account the possibility that x_2 could be related to $b_{1.2}$, and similarly in the second equation x_1 could be related to $b_{2.1}$. It is clearly the δ's that allow this to happen, and assuming both δ's are zero is CIFC - *conditional independence of factors and co-causes*. Without the δ's, each factor is conditionally independent of the co-cause of the other factor, or

$$b_{1.2} \perp\!\!\!\perp x_2 \,|x_1=1, b_{0.12}=0$$

$$b_{2.1} \perp\!\!\!\perp x_1 \,|x_2=1, b_{0.12}=0 \quad \text{CIFC}$$

The next equation is the most difficult to decipher:

$$P[b_{1.2}\vee b_{2.1}=1|x_1=1,x_2=1,b_{0.12}=0] = \beta_{1.2} \vee \delta_{2.1} \vee \beta_{2.1} \vee \delta_{1.2} \vee \delta_{12}$$

The first thing to note here is that the first two terms on the right are the conditional probability that $b_{1.2}=1$ given $x_1=x_2=1$ and $b_{0.12}=0$, and there is a similar observation for the second pair. Now going back to Section 5 where I introduced the $\vee$-notation, the above equation can actually be seen to define δ_{12} as the measure of negative dependence between $b_{1.2}$ and $b_{2.1}$, conditioning on the events behind the bar. Assuming that $\delta_{12}=0$ is CICC - *conditional independence of co-causes*, and is equivalent to

$b_{1.2} \amalg b_{2.1} | x_1=1, x_2=1, b_{0.12}=0$ CICC

Let us now go back and assume that all of the δ's may be present. By systematically using the rules that I introduced in Section 5, we can find that

$P[y=1|x_1,x_2] =$

$\beta_{0.12} \vee (\beta_{1.2} \vee \delta_{0.1.2}) x_1 \vee (\beta_{2.1} \vee \delta_{0.2.1}) x_2 \vee (\beta_{12} \vee \delta_{0.12} \vee \delta_{1.2} \vee \delta_{2.1} \vee \delta_{12}) x_1 x_2$

To do this, first compute

$P[y=1|x_1,x_2] = P[b_{0.12}=1|x_1,x_2] \vee P[b_{1.2}x_1 \vee b_{2.1}x_2 \vee b_{12}x_1x_2=1|x_1,x_2,b_{0.12}=0]$

and note that the first term on the right is

$\beta_{0.12} \vee \delta_{0.1.2} x_1 \vee \delta_{0.2.1} x_2 \vee \delta_{0.12} x_1 x_2$

The second term on the right is

$P[b_{1.2}x_1 \vee b_{2.1}x_2=1|x_1,x_2,b_{0.12}=0] \vee P[b_{12}x_1x_2=1|b_{1.2}x_1 \vee b_{2.1}x_2=0 \; x_1,x_2,b_{0.12}=0]$

The term at the right of this expression is

$P[b_{12}=1|b_{1.2} \vee b_{2.1}=0, x_1=1, x_2=1, b_{0.12}=0] = \beta_{12}$

Since $b_{1.2}x_1 \amalg b_{2.1}x_2 | x_1,x_2,b_{0.12}=0$, the term on the left one expression back is

$P[b_{1.2}=1|x_1=1,x_2,b_{0.12}=0]x_1 \vee P[b_{2.1}=1|x_1,x_2=1,b_{0.12}=0]x_2$

$= (\beta_{1.2} \vee \delta_{2.1}x_2)x_1 \vee (\beta_{2.1} \vee \delta_{1.2}x_1)x_2$

Since the x's are factors, we can use the distributive rule to collect terms. This completes the demonstration of the complete model formula.

Contrast the complete model formula with the equation that we would like to hold, in which all of the δ's are zero:

$P[y=1|x_1,x_2] = \beta_{0.12} \vee \beta_{1.2}x_1 \vee \beta_{2.1}x_2 \vee \beta_{12}x_1x_2$

I like this latter equation, for at least two reasons. First, it perfectly mirrors the causal structural equation. Secondly, each β parameter has a clear causal interpretation. $\beta_{0.12}$ measures the presence of residual causes, unconfounded with whether or not x_1 or x_2 occurred. $\beta_{1.2}$ represents the causal force of x_1, unconfounded with whether x_2 occurred or not. Similarly for $\beta_{2.1}$. Finally, β_{12} represents the causal force of the pathway x_1x_2, unconfounded by any association between the x's and the residual cause, unconfounded by any relationships between each x and the co-cause of the other x, and unconfounded by negative dependence between the co-causes.

I use the term "unconfounded" here because it is the word that has become common in epidemiology for describing this situation. I would prefer, however, to say that in the last equation above, the β's were *correctly specified*. In other words, saying that the causal effects I am interested in were correctly specified in the model means just that the δ's that might make them incorrectly specified are zero. In yet other words, go back two equations and see that the following conditions will correctly specify each β.

Causal Parameter	Assumed zero
$\beta_{1.2}$	$\delta_{0.1.2}$
$\beta_{2.1}$	$\delta_{0.2.1}$
β_{12}	$\delta_{0.12}, \delta_{1.2}, \delta_{2.1}, \delta_{12}$

Clearly IFR is important, because it potentially affects all three parameters. CIFC and CICC are both necessary to make β_{12} correctly specified.

If we have a model in which all of the causal parameters are correctly specified, then we can solve for them trivially

$$\beta_{0.12} = P[y=1|x_1=0,x_2=0]$$

$$\beta_{1.2} = P[y=1|x_1=1,x_2=0] \setminus P[y=1|x_1=0,x_2=0]$$

$$\beta_{2.1} = P[y=1|x_1=0,x_2=1] \setminus P[y=1|x_1=0,x_2=0]$$

$$\beta_{12} = P[y=1|x_1=1,x_2=1] \setminus P[y=1|x_1=1,x_2=0] \setminus$$

$$P[y=1|x_1=0,x_2=1] \vee P[y=1|x_1=0,x_2=0]$$

In the unfortunate situation where one or more of the β's are mis-specified, these equations are wrong.

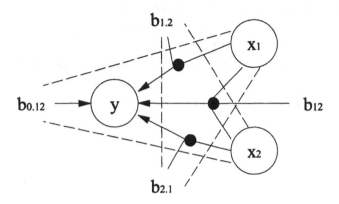

Figure 1. The two-factor causal model, with dashed lines showing the unwanted relationships.

There are some very important lessons from this section. They are fairly apparent in the two-factor case, and they hint at even more complex problems in the multi-factor case. The basic idea is to define parameters that measure the causal effects of the b-factors that appear in the causal structural equation. Because factors can be probabilistically related, we need to take into account potential relationships between x-causes and residual causes, between x-causes and b-co-causes, and between b-co-causes themselves. As we have seen, all of these stochastic relationships are possible, and they frustrate the attempt to get at the causal parameters.

These considerations are not trivial. They suggest that studies trying to uncover causal relationships when two or more factors are involved, may have a difficult time unless they essentially identify all of the major causal factors, so that the influences that mis-specify causal parameters will become small. One might take this to be rather alarming in the light of the modern trend to try to isolate the causal effects of single factors, and the corresponding prejudice against finding interaction terms, which correspond to joint pathways involving two or more factors. If the MSC approach to causation is at all accurate, then there is perhaps not so much mystery about why we have difficulty understanding complex causal systems.

This is particularly troubling with regard to the β_{12} parameter. This is intended to capture the force of joint pathways that involve both x_1 and x_2, but a rather large number of the δ's can cause mis-specification of this parameter. One suspects that many studies finding no "interaction" or a "contradictory interaction" are in fact experiencing mis-specification.

Down Syndrome Example

Down syndrome is a genetic affliction of newborn babies. Although life expectancy has increased, there are still a substantial number of deaths in the first ten years. The data in Table 1 show survival and five factors that might be causes of survival.

We can consider these data from several perspectives. First, we think of the sample as a population, and compute the minimal sufficient causes. Here is the computer output:

```
====== Minimal Sufficient Cause ======
Effect=alive
Causes=s a c p v
Explanation   Exception    Non-Miss   Cause
-----------   ---------    --------   -----
   5(0.045)   0(0.000)  148(1.000)    s a
  22(0.200)   0(0.000)  148(1.000)    s p
   9(0.082)   0(0.000)  148(1.000)    s v
   2(0.018)   0(0.000)  148(1.000)    a c
-----------   ---------    --------   -----
  27(0.245)
```

First of all $C[alive|F] = 1$ occurs in 27 cases, which was 0.245 of all those who lived. It is implicit here that $F = \{s, a, c, p, v\}$. This indicates that many of the survivals are not explained by these factors alone. The minimal sufficient causes themselves were sa, sp sv, and ac. The extreme left of each row shows how many occurrences each minimal sufficient cause explained. We can now write

$$C[alive|F] = ac \vee (a \vee p \vee v)s \quad causal[F]$$

showing the residual cause and co-cause with respect to s. If we were interested in s and a as causes, then we would write the same equation as

$$C[alive|F] = (p \vee v)s \vee (c)a \vee sa \qquad causal[F]$$

In this case, there is no residual cause, there are only pathways involving s, a, and sa. Obviously, we could factor this in a number of other ways, to highlight the roles of other factors, or pairs of factors. We can also consider complementing some of the factors. For example, if $F = \{a, c, p, v, v^*\}$ then

a	c	p	v	s	alive	num
0	0	0	0	0	1	0
0	0	0	0	0	0	0
0	0	0	0	1	1	1
0	0	0	0	1	0	0
0	0	0	1	0	1	26
0	0	0	1	0	0	4
0	0	0	1	1	1	1
0	0	0	1	1	0	0
0	0	1	0	0	1	7
0	0	1	0	0	0	1
0	0	1	0	1	1	8
0	0	1	0	1	0	0
0	0	1	1	0	1	5
0	0	1	1	0	0	1
0	0	1	1	1	1	5
0	0	1	1	1	0	0
0	1	0	0	0	1	19
0	1	0	0	0	0	22
0	1	0	0	1	1	6
0	1	0	0	1	0	2
0	1	0	1	0	1	0
0	1	0	1	0	0	0
0	1	0	1	1	1	0
0	1	0	1	1	0	0
0	1	1	0	0	1	1
0	1	1	0	0	0	2
0	1	1	0	1	1	7
0	1	1	0	1	0	0
0	1	1	1	0	1	0
0	1	1	1	0	0	0
0	1	1	1	1	1	0
0	1	1	1	1	0	0
1	0	0	0	0	1	8
1	0	0	0	0	0	2
1	0	0	0	1	1	0
1	0	0	0	1	0	0
1	0	0	1	0	1	8
1	0	0	1	0	0	3
1	0	0	1	1	1	2
1	0	0	1	1	0	0
1	0	1	0	0	1	2
1	0	1	0	0	0	0
1	0	1	0	1	1	1
1	0	1	0	1	0	0
1	0	1	1	0	1	0
1	0	1	1	0	0	1
1	0	1	1	1	1	1
1	0	1	1	1	0	0
1	1	0	0	0	1	0
1	1	0	0	0	0	0
1	1	0	0	1	1	1
1	1	0	0	1	0	0
1	1	0	1	0	1	0
1	1	0	1	0	0	0
1	1	0	1	1	1	0
1	1	0	1	1	0	0
1	1	1	0	0	1	1
1	1	1	0	0	0	0
1	1	1	0	1	1	0
1	1	1	0	1	0	0
1	1	1	1	0	1	0
1	1	1	1	0	0	0
1	1	1	1	1	1	0
1	1	1	1	1	0	0

Table 1 (previous page). a = atrio-septal defects, c = complete atrio-septal defect, p = patent ductus arteriosis, v = ventral septal defect, s = surgery, alive = survival to age ten, num = number of children. (International Journal of Epidemiology 1997;26:822-829)

$$C[y|F] = apv^* \vee (a)c \vee (a \vee p \vee v)s \qquad causal[F]$$

highlights c and s as causes. Here we have a residual cause, but no co-cause of sc, indicating no joint causal pathway.

Note that in these cases, each of the defect factors really means "this defect, as opposed to some other". We might ask, if we turn the defects around and use only their complements, what do we get? Here is the output:

```
====== Minimal Sufficient Cause ======
Effect=alive
Causes=s a* c* p* v*
Explanation   Exception   Non-Miss   Cause
-----------   ---------   --------   -----
 19(0.173)    0(0.000)   148(1.000)  s c*
  1(0.009)    0(0.000)   148(1.000)  a* c* p* v*
-----------   ---------   --------   -----
 19(0.173)
```

This explains fewer survivals, and provides a less interesting equation, somewhat surprisingly.

Another question we can ask is whether the type of defect might cause surgery. Since the study from which these data were extracted was not a trial, surgery was not an intervention, but rather it was elected as it normally is. It turns out that there are no minimal sufficient causes of surgery. This might only indicate, of course, that there are other factors, which we have not observed, that also play causal roles. Thus, it would be reasonable to estimate the causal parameters:

$$P[s=1|p,v] = 0.16 \vee 0.44p \vee (-0.11)v \vee (-0.04)pv$$

The values are the maximum likelihood estimates. It is not a contradiction that some are negative, since what counts is that the entire expression on the right side is between 0 and 1. Nevertheless, with a causal system the causal parameters theoretically cannot drop below zero, and this suggests that we change the causal field:

$$P[s=1|p,v^*] = 0.07 \vee 0.42p \vee 0.10v^* \vee 0.03pv^*$$

The joint coefficient 0.03 is only 1/10 of its sampling standard deviation, and so it would usually be dropped from the equation, giving essentially the same result

$$P[s=1|p,v^*] = 0.07 \vee 0.43p \vee 0.10v^*$$

Of all the equations that one can fit, this actually appears to be one of the better ones. Thus, the indication is that p (patent ductus arteriosis) and v* (absence of ventral septal defect) might play some role in causing election of surgery, but most likely the other two factors play no role.

When I started out this example, note that I considered the sample to be the population. This made the computation of minimal sufficient causes more interesting, because it allowed me to say something about occurrences that were completely explained. It is inevitable, however, that some of the questions one wants to ask (like, what causes surgery?) are going to require theory and measurements beyond what we have. In these cases, we will usually want to estimate causal parameters, because we want to reason in some sense from the sample we have to the population it represents.

In estimating parameters, one generally ignores the mis-specification problem. This is not because it is unimportant, but because there is usually no evidence about the unwanted δ parameters. In this case, I am reasonably sure that information about δ's is not contained in the factors I left out of the final equation (a and c), since neither they, their product, nor their products with p or v* had much effect on the coefficient estimates for these latter two factors in the final equation. This does not prove that the equation is correct, but it provides at least some support. It is, of course, perfectly possible that there is a factor not in the data which, when entered into the model, would render both p and v* causally irrelevant.

14

Marginalization

Suppose that we have the causal relationship

$$b_{0.12} \lor b_{1.2}x_1 \lor b_{2.1}x_2 \lor b_{12}x_1x_2 \xrightarrow{s} y \quad [\mathbf{F}]$$

Clearly, at the same time we have another causal relationship

$$b_{0.1} \lor b_1 x_1 \xrightarrow{s} y \quad [\mathbf{F}]$$

In this section I want to study the relationship between these two relationships. As usual, I assume $\longrightarrow$ is MSC.

The first result is

$$b_{0.1} = b_{0.12} \lor b_{2.1}x_2 \quad \text{causal}[\mathbf{F}_1]$$

Here is the demonstration. The first part follows from a fact that is interesting on its own:

$$\text{if } \mathbf{G} \subseteq \mathbf{F}, \text{ then } C[C[y|\mathbf{F}]|\mathbf{G}] = C[y|\mathbf{G}]$$

This follows from the facts that for any $f \in \Pi\mathbf{G}$, $f \xrightarrow{NT} C[y|\mathbf{G}] \Leftrightarrow f \xrightarrow{s} y \Leftrightarrow f \xrightarrow{s} C[y|\mathbf{F}] \Leftrightarrow f \xrightarrow{NT} C[C[y|\mathbf{F}]|\mathbf{G}]$. To apply this to the result we are demonstrating, $C[b_{0.1}|\mathbf{F}_{12}] = C[C[y|\mathbf{F}_1]|\mathbf{F}_{12}] = C[y|\mathbf{F}_{12}]$. This shows that $b_{0.12}$ is the residual cause. For the rest of the demonstration, for any $f \in \Pi\mathbf{F}_{12}$, $f \xrightarrow{s} b_{0.1} \Leftrightarrow f \xrightarrow{s} y$, and since $fx_2 \in \Pi\mathbf{F}_1$, $fx_2 \xrightarrow{s} b_{0.1} \Leftrightarrow fx_2 \xrightarrow{s} y$. This shows that the definition of the co-cause of x_2 as a cause of $b_{0.1}$ coincides with the definition of $b_{2.1}$. This completes the demonstration.

Recall that the verbal interpretation of $b_{0.1}$ is that it is all the causes of y (generated by $\mathbf{F}$) that can be constructed without reference to x_1. The result demonstrated above adds some depth to this interpretation, by showing that $b_{0.1}$ is composed of $b_{0.12}$, those causes that can be constructed without referring to either x_1 or x_2, and $b_{2.1}x_2$, the causes due to x_2 but not x_1. The fact that this equation is causal is very nice.

The corresponding result for the co-cause is algebraically satisfying, but not generally causal:

$$b_1 = b_{1.2} \vee b_{12} x_2$$

To demonstrate this, first note that every f in the definition of $b_{1.2}$ is also in the definition of b_1. Further, if f appears in the definition of b_{12}, then $fx_2 \in \Pi F_1$ and $fx_2 \overset{\rightarrow}{\rightarrow} y$ imply that fx_2 is in the definition of b_1. This shows that $b_1 \geq b_{1.2} \vee b_{12} x_2$. Conversely, suppose that f is in the definition of b_1. If $f \in \Pi F_{12}$, then f is in the definition of $b_{1.2}$. Otherwise, if $f = gx_2$ with $g \in \Pi F_{12}$ then either g is in the definition of b_{12} implying $f \leq b_{12} x_2$, or else $gx_1 \overset{\rightarrow}{\rightarrow} y$ implying g in the definition of $b_{1.2}$ because $g \overset{\rightarrow}{\rightarrow} y$. This shows that $b_1 \leq b_{1.2} \vee b_{12} x_2$, completing the demonstration.

Recalling that b_1 was interpreted as the disjunction of all pathways not referring to x_1, but together with x_1 sufficient for y, this latter result goes a few steps further to identify the components of b_1 as $b_{1.2}$, the complementary pathways not referring to either x_1 or x_2, and $b_{12} x_2$, the complementary pathways that do refer to x_2.

With these results in hand, we are prepared to answer an important inferential question; should we use the marginal model (with x_1 as a single factor) or the joint model (with x_1 and x_2 as factors) to analyze our data? One reason this seems a reasonably query is that the marginal model seems to require less (only the IFR) for its parameters to be correctly specified. The joint model requires not only IFR, but also CIFR and CICC. Does this suggest that the marginal model is to be preferred?

To answer this question, we need to consider the conditions under which the marginal IFR will hold, from the standpoint of the joint parametrization. The first step is to compute

$$P[b_{0.1}=1|x_1,x_2] = P[b_{0.12} \vee b_{2.1} x_2=1|x_1,x_2] =$$

$$=P[b_{0.12}=1|x_1,x_2] \vee P[b_{2.1} x_2=1|x_1,x_2,b_{0.12}=0]=$$

$$=\beta_{0.12} \vee \delta_{0.1.2} x_1 \vee (\beta_{2.1} \vee \delta_{0.2.1}) x_2 \vee (\delta_{1.2} \vee \delta_{0.12}) x_1 x_2$$

Let us now introduce new parameters for

$$P[x_2=1|x_1] = \xi_0 \vee \xi_1 x_1$$

It follows that

$$P[b_{0.1}=1|x_1] = \beta_{0.12} \vee \delta_{0.1.2} x_1 \vee \{\beta_{2.1} \vee \delta_{0.2.1} \vee (\delta_{1.2} \vee \delta_{0.12}) x_1\} (\xi_0 \vee \xi_1 x_1)$$

Now recall that the marginal IFR states that this latter expression does not depend on x_1. This is equivalent to

$$(\beta_{2.1} \vee \delta_{0.2.1})\xi_0 = \delta_{0.1.2} \vee (\beta_{2.1} \vee \delta_{0.2.1} \vee \delta_{1.2} \vee \delta_{0.12})(\xi_0 \vee \xi_1)$$

No doubt there are many parameter combinations that will make this true, but it seems rather clear that the only unartificial case is

$$\delta_{0.2.1} = \delta_{0.1.2} = \delta_{0.12} = \delta_{1.2} = \xi_1 = 0$$

We could, of course, easily exempt $\delta_{0.2.1}$ from this list. Then we would have the joint IFR (except maybe for $\delta_{0.2.1}$), part of the CIFC, and $x_1 \perp\!\!\!\perp x_2$.

The answer to our question seems fairly clear. The marginal IFR is not simpler than the joint IFR, and in fact, generally one would expect to have to assume all of the joint IFR (except perhaps $\delta_{0.2.1}=0$), part of the CIFC, and most stringently, independence of x_1 and x_2, in order for the marginal IFR to hold. This result suggests a possible generalization; the more factors included in the model, the fewer the assumptions necessary for correct specification of causal parameters.

Let us now make the natural assumptions given at the top if this page. Then we have

$$\beta_{0.1} = \beta_{0.12} \vee \beta_{2.1}\xi_0$$

an equation that fits nicely with

$$b_{0.1} = b_{0.12} \vee b_{2.1}x_2$$

Turning to the computation of the marginal causal effect,

$$\beta_1 = P[b_{1.2} \vee b_{12}x_2 | x_1=1, b_{0.1}=0] =$$

$$= P[b_{1.2}=1 | x_1=1, x_2=0, b_{0.12}=0]\xi_0^* +$$

$$+ P[b_{1.2} \vee b_{12}=1 | x_1=1, x_2=1, b_{0.12}=0, b_{2.1}=0]\xi_0$$

$$= \beta_{1.2}\xi_0^* + (\beta_{1(2)} \vee \beta_{12})\xi_0$$

Here, the new parameter $\beta_{1(2)}$ signifies the potential failure of CICC. When CICC holds, the above reduces to

$$\beta_1 = \beta_{1.2} \vee (\beta_{12} \vee \delta_{2.1})\xi_0$$

89

We must thus assume the other half of CIFC in order to obtain the model equation

$$\beta_1 = \beta_{1.2} \vee \beta_{12} \xi_0$$

that nicely parallels the mathematical equation

$$b_1 = b_{0.1} \vee b_{12} x_2$$

The conclusion from all of these computations is that the marginal model is not, in some sense, simpler than the joint model. In order for any reasonable degree of causal parameter specification in the marginal model, virtually all of the joint IFR, CIFC, and CICC must hold, and in addition x_1 and x_2 must be independent. The end result is that there are probably not any realistic circumstances in which the marginal model would be preferable if the joint model were available.

Stratification

In the preceding section I considered how I could focus on the factor of interest by ignoring a second factor. In this section I investigate the opposite situation, in which I take the second factor into consideration to the maximum degree. The basic assumption in this section is that for the MSC causation $\longrightarrow$ I have the causal relationship

$$b_{0.12} \vee b_{1.2}x_1 \vee b_{2.1}x_2 \vee b_{12}x_1x_2 \rightarrow y \quad [\mathbf{F}]$$

Here x_1 is the factor I am most interested in.

Stratification means breaking this relationship into two pieces, depending on the value of x_2:

$$b_{0.12} \vee b_{1.2}x_1 \rightarrow y \quad [\mathbf{F}] \text{ on } [x_2=0]$$

$$b_{0.12} \vee b_{2.1} \vee (b_{1.2} \vee b_{12})x_1 \rightarrow y \quad [\mathbf{F}] \text{ on } [x_2=1]$$

I presume that the causation has the property that causal relationships in the population persist in subpopulations, such as the two specified above.

The first issue is the IFR in the two subpopulations. On $[x_2=0]$ we have

$$P[b_{0.12}=1|x_1,x_2=0] = \beta_{0.12} \vee \delta_{0.1.2}x_1$$

while on $[x_2=1]$ we have

$$P[b_{0.12} \vee b_{2.1}=1|x_1,x_2=1] = \beta_{0.12} \vee \delta_{0.2.1} \vee \beta_{2.1} \vee (\delta_{0.1.2} \vee \delta_{0.12} \vee \delta_{1.2})x_1$$

For IFR in the first subpopulation, I need $\delta_{0.1.2}=0$. For IFR in the second subpopulation, I need $\delta_{0.1.2} \vee \delta_{0.12} \vee \delta_{1.2}=0$. While there are multiple values of the individual parameters that will make this happen, they seem rather strained, and the natural condition is that they are all zero. So let us assume the joint IFR and part of CIFC in order to obtain the stratified IFR's.

We can now compute

$$P[b_{1.2}=1|x_1=1,x_2=0,b_{0.12}=0] = \beta_{1.2}$$

$$P[b_{1.2} \vee b_{12}=1|x_1=1, x_2=1, b_{0.12} \vee b_{2.1}=0] = \beta_{1(2)} \vee \beta_{12}$$

where the new parameter $\beta_{1(2)}$ signifies possible failure of CICC. If we assume CICC then $\beta_{1(2)}$ becomes $\beta_{1.2}$ and we have

$$P[b_1=1|x_1=1, x_2, b_{0.1}=0] = \beta_{1.2} \vee \beta_{12}x_2$$

In this derivation, I could have allowed $\delta_{0.2.1}$ to be non-zero, but I essentially had to assume the remainder of the IFR. Likewise, I had to assume only half of the CIFC, but all of the CICC.

It is worthwhile to step back and put this and the preceding section together. In presentations that argue for a stratified analysis, the first step is to exhibit a joint model in which the parameter of interest can be unambiguously identified. In our case, this would likely be $\beta_{1.2}$, although it would seem that β_{12} might also be of interest. The development then shows that $\beta_{1.2}$ is mis-specified in the marginal analysis. The culprit here is usually identified as a stochastic relationship between x_1 and x_2. The demonstration then turns to the stratified analysis, showing that $\beta_{1.2}$ is correctly specified.

In causal models, there are several problems with this line of reasoning. There is no problem rejecting the marginal model, since we have seen that it requires essentially the joint IFR, CIFC and CICC, plus independence of x_1 and x_2. Where the standard development fails is in claiming that since the marginal model is so bad, and the stratified model is better, we should use the stratified model, ignoring the possibility of a third alternative superior to both. As we have seen, the stratified model itself requires nearly all of the joint IFR, CIFC, and CICC, in order for the causal parameters to be correctly specified. Moreover, as the last equation above shows, any estimate of the x_1 effect (putatively $\beta_{1.2}$) that comes from the two stratified analyses will be mis-specified if there are joint pathways, since then $\beta_{12} \neq 0$. So we have to assume no joint pathways to get $\beta_{1.2}$ correctly specified in the stratified models.

Since both the marginal and stratified models require virtually all of the IFR, CIFC, and CICC, for the correct specification of parameters, and since they each require an additional condition (independence or lack of joint pathways) to be sensible procedures, it would seem reasonable to take the position that they are both flawed. Indeed, if one were willing to make even a fraction of the assumptions required by these inferential strategies, it would seem that the joint model would be the preferred method. In other words, it is hard to see when either the marginal or stratified analyses would be better than the joint analysis.

To see this in an application, consider the Down syndrome example. First we estimate the joint model

$$P[\text{alive}=1|s,c*] = 0.47 \lor 0.77s \lor 0.67c* \lor sc*$$

The fitted marginal model is

$$P[\text{alive}=1|s] = 0.68 \lor 0.82s$$

while the fitted stratified models are

$$P[\text{alive}=1|s] = 0.47 \lor 0.77s \quad \text{on } [c*=0]$$

$$P[\text{alive}=1|s] = 0.82 \lor s \quad \text{on } [c*=1]$$

It seems clear that the marginal model is not a gross distortion, but of course the reason this happened in this particular case is that it is reasonable to believe that s and c* are independent (p=0.5 by the usual chi-square test). The stratified analysis is, however, quite misleading, since it suggests that the effect we should attribute to s is some combination of 0.77 and 1.0. The joint model makes the situation obvious. In particular, it uncovers the interesting fact that in the sample sc* is a sufficient cause. Of course, additional sampling might well destroy this perfect result, but one could nevertheless expect the resulting β_{12} to be close to 1.0. This is an example of the kind of joint pathway discovery that is one of the benefits of using the joint model. In this case, trying to find a "real" estimate of the force of s seems rather silly if the sc* pathway has the strongest causal force that is present in the joint model.

Many of the arguments that have been given in the literature to support various inferential strategies have been unmotivated by any underlying notion of causation. This leaves them with heuristic or rhetorical illustrations, but little else. This is not to say that no one will ever find a causal rationale for them, just that no one has so far. The minimal sufficient cause approach agrees with conventional wisdom in saying beware of marginal models. It departs from conventional wisdom in saying also beware of stratified models. The information in the several and joint causal pathways is contained in the joint model, which is the model that should be used for analysis.

Obesity Example

In this section I want to consider some data relating gender and physical activity to obesity, shown in Table 1. I am going to approach this as though gender and inactivity are causes of obesity. It is worth noting, however, that even if this is wrong, there is little or no harm in performing the analysis as if it were correct. Causal models are also associational models, so that those who do not want to make causal interpretations can fail to do so. The reverse is not the case, since most associational models are not causal, so that the use of a purely associational model can prevent a causal interpretation.

Physical Activity	Gender	Obese
None	Male	14/69 = .203
	Female	5/48 = .104
Some	Male	127/888 = .143
	Female	125/921 = .136

Annals of Epidemiology 1998;8(7):422-432

Table 1. Data relating gender and physical activity to obesity among teenagers.

To make this example correspond to preceding notation, let us take y = obesity, x_1 = inactivity, x_2 = male. Assuming that the causal parameters are correctly specified, we compute

$\beta_{0.12} = 0.136$

$\beta_{1.2} = 0.104 \setminus 0.136 = -0.037$

$\beta_{2.1} = 0.143 \setminus 0.136 = 0.008$

$\beta_{12} = 0.203 \setminus 0.104 \setminus 0.143 \vee 0.136 = 0.103$

Thus, the estimated causal equation is

P[obese=1|male,inact] =

$= 0.136 \vee (-0.037)\text{inact} \vee 0.008\text{male} \vee 0.103(\text{male})(\text{inact})$

Without belaboring the obvious, the most striking fact is the size of the effect of the joint pathway. There is virtually no pathway including maleness without inactivity, and if anything the pathways involving inactivity without maleness have the wrong sign. This can mean either that sampling variability has given us a negative value when the true parameter is zero, or it might mean that we need to modify the overall model to allow "inactivity* $\longrightarrow$ obesity".

The points that I would like to make with this example do not require me to change the basic model. I would like to consider what would happen in this analysis, if I were to ignore the male factor, and moreover I would like to see what happens in terms of the joint causal parameters. To do this, I first need the model equation

$P[\text{male}=1|\text{inact}] = \beta_{2:0.1} \vee \beta_{2:1}\text{inact}$

Note here that the number before the colon (:) indicates the effect variable, and those after the colon follow the same pattern I have used before. I will use this notation when there are multiple causal equations involving the same set of variables.

By direct computation

P[male=1|inact=0] = 0.491

P[male=1|inact=1] = 0.590

and so

$P[\text{male}=1|\text{inact}] = 0.491 \vee 0.194\text{inact}$

The situation so far can be summarized in the causal diagram of Figure 1, where the male/inact relationship is just associational.

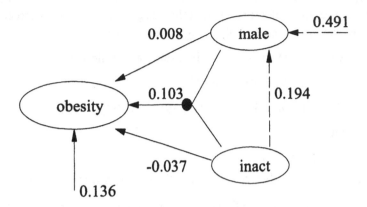

Figure 1. Causal diagram for the obesity example,
showing path coefficients.

The principle that allows us to figure out how the joint parameters
relate to the marginal parameters is

$$P[A|B] = P[AC|B]+P[AC^*|B] =$$

$$= P[A|CB]P[C|B]+ P[A|C^*B]P[C^*|B]$$

The first line is because probability measures are additive, and the second
consists of two applications of the chain rule. Thus we can compute

$$P[y=1|x_1] = P[y=1|x_1,x_2=0]P[x_2=0|x_1]$$

$$+ P[y=1|x_1,x_2=1]P[x_2=1|x_1]$$

$$= (\beta_{0.12}\vee\beta_{1.2}x_1)(\beta_{2:0.1}\vee\beta_{2:1}x_1)^*$$

$$+(\beta_{0.12}\vee\beta_{1.2}x_1\vee\beta_{2.1}\vee\beta_{12}x_1)(\beta_{2:0.1}\vee\beta_{2:1}x_1)$$

$$= \beta_{0.12}\vee\beta_{1.2}x_1\vee(\beta_{2.1}\vee\beta_{12}x_1)(\beta_{2:0.1}\vee\beta_{2:1}x_1)$$

Inspecting this formula, we can see

$$\beta_{0.1} \sim \beta_{0.12}\vee\beta_{2.1}\beta_{2:0.1}$$

$$\beta_1 \sim \beta_{1.2}\vee(\beta_{2.1}\vee\beta_{12})(\beta_{2:0.1}\vee\beta_{2:1}) \setminus \beta_{2.1}\beta_{2:0.1}$$

The wiggle sign ($\sim$) means the right side "is supposed to correspond to"
the left side. That is, when we use the marginal model, we want to have
estimates of the two parameters at the left, but in the circumstance where
only the joint model is correctly specified, our marginal model will

actually get the expressions on the right for the parameters on the left. What one would hope, of course, is that the marginal model were correctly specified as well, in which case the ~ signs would turn into equalities.

We can verify these equations in the example as follows:

$\beta_{0.1} \sim 0.136 \vee (0.008)(0.491) = 0.139$

$\beta_1 \sim -0.037 \vee (0.008 \vee 0.103)(0.491 \vee 0.194) \setminus (0.008)(0.491)$

$\quad = 0.027$

If we were to directly compute the causal parameters for the one-factor model "inactivity $\longrightarrow$ obesity", these are the numbers we would get.

Now the conclusion would be that inactivity is a cause of obesity, although perhaps only a weak one. Looking at the expression for β_1 in terms of the joint parameters, we see that it is $\beta_{1.2}$, which is presumably what we want, $\vee$-plus some more stuff. This additional stuff will generally vanish only when $x_1 \amalg x_2$, so that $\beta_{2.1} = 0$, and there are no joint pathways, so $\beta_{12} = 0$. In our case neither of these hold, There is a positive association between inactivity and male, and there are joint pathways.

This example is important for several reasons. First, it illustrates the methods by which we can investigate how some parameters (the marginal ones in this case) relate to others (the joint ones in this case). This provides a powerful tool for discussing the threats to validity in a research study. If it does nothing else, the causal perspective should provide a language for talking about these threats, and assessing where they reside.

Secondly, the obesity example points up how misinformative marginal models can be. In this case a relatively strong joint pathways effect would have been interpreted as an independent effect of inactivity. Now to be sure, there is a causal effect of inactivity in this model, but the crucial point is that it pertains to pathways that are joint with maleness. By considering the marginal model alone we lose this information, and we also see a reduction in the magnitude of the effect.

A very common strategy in analyzing disease/risk factor associations in epidemiology and public health is to look for "main effects" (corresponding to $\beta_{1.2}$ and $\beta_{2.1}$) and to ignore or downplay "interaction effects" (corresponding to β_{12}). When researchers find large main effects then they say that they have established an "independent" effect of the factor under consideration, and if the frequency with which this happens in the literature is any guide, one would judge that it is something to be prized. As the obesity example makes clear, the "independent" effect of inactivity more than likely represents joint pathways with factors not considered (as maleness is not considered in the marginal model). In other words, the emphasis on the search for an "independent effect" means that it is considered more important to find pathways involving the factor of interest and other factors not included in the study, than it is to find pathways involving the factor of interest and other factors that were included in the study. The MSC approach provides very little support for this conventional analytic method.

The obesity example illustrates a third lesson. It is virtually a cliché in biomedical research that the only way to establish causation is through a randomized trial. There is an entire menu of reasons why this is supposed to be true, but one key argument is that by assigning the "treatment" at random, it is made independent of all other potential causal factors, and this removes the problem with using marginal models. As a consequence, it is almost always argued that marginal models are appropriate in randomized studies, and that they are unique in giving the correct, causal effect.

Suppose, therefore, that the obesity model is causally correct, insofar as it tells how maleness and inactivity cause obesity. Further suppose that we carry out a trial in which physical inactivity is assigned at random, and the teenagers in the study are then followed-up for several years. Suppose lastly that all of the usual problems of such trials are absent, so that there are no additional sources of mis-specification. Under all of these conditions, the marginal effect is

$$\beta_1 \sim \beta_{1.2} \vee (\beta_{2:0.1} \setminus \beta_{2.1}\beta_{2:0.1})\beta_{12}$$

This follows from the equation I derived above, with some unitary algebraic manipulation, and using the fact that male is now unrelated to inactivity ($\beta_{2:1}=0$). Substituting the estimates:

$$\beta_1 \sim -0.037 \vee (0.491 \setminus (0.008)(0.491))(0.103) = 0.015$$

This is not $\beta_{1.2}$, so I have not captured the causal pathways that are unique to inactivity. It is also far from β_{12}, so I have missed the joint pathways with maleness. By not including maleness in the model (which the

99

randomization philosophy says I was supposed to leave out) I have failed to even see the possibility of these joint pathways.

The defenders of randomization will point out that I have made very strong causal assumptions, and that I have not considered the potential roles of other important factors. They will then go on to enumerate how randomization will resolve problems that I have merely assumed away. This is the sort of argument that people must deal with if they have the temerity to criticize the view that randomization is a panacea. What the argument ignores, of course, is that if my scenario were correct, then randomization has failed. Not only that, but the example shows why it fails - because we cannot make x_1 independent of x_1x_2 by randomization or any other means.

What I think this shows is that the arguments favoring randomization succeed only by ruling out the kinds of problems that randomization cannot solve. Arguments against randomization often suffer the same defect in reverse. The important point is that a causal approach, and in specific the MSC approach, provides a context, a language, and examples that can be used to shed light on this important issue in the design of research studies.

Attribution

It could be argued that one of the main reasons for having an idea of causation in the first place is to be able to explain why certain events happen. If causal rules are laws that nature has to obey, then even if we don't understand why nature must operate under these constraints, we feel that an occurrence which follows from a comprehensible causal system has been explained.

There is a natural desire to want to go further than this, and to find in a given case whether a specific factor was a cause of the observed effect *in that particular instance*. This is the notion of singular causation that I introduced in Section 3 and discussed in Section 6, where I said that nontrivial implication will often give unsatisfying answers. One of the themes of this section is that one cannot generally expect any MSC causation to solve the singular causation problem.

To see an example, let us (as usual) assume that $\longrightarrow$ is an MSC causation. Suppose we have

$$C[y|\mathbf{F}] = b_{0.1} \vee b_1 x_1 \qquad \text{causal}[\mathbf{F}]$$

The right side can be re-written as

$$(b_{0.1} \backslash b_1 x_1) \vee b_{0.1} b_1 x_1 \vee (b_1 x_1 \backslash b_{0.1})$$

The first term in parentheses can easily be interpreted as all cases in which factors other than x_1 caused y, because $b_1 x_1$ consists of all pathways in which x_1 is a necessary part of the cause, and it is not present. Similarly, the other term in parentheses can be interpreted as those cases where x_1 was part of the cause, because $b_{0.1}$ consists of all pathways in which x_1 is not mentioned, and $b_{0.1}$ is not present. The middle term is ambiguous, since one could attribute the cause either to x_1 (since $b_1 x_1$ is present) or to factors unrelated to x_1 (since $b_{0.1}$ is present). There is no way to resolve the ambiguity of the middle term.

We can expect this kind of ambiguity to arise frequently, and it may happen even when we are considering a rather large number of explanatory factors (x's). It is simply in the nature of things that some people will exhibit two or more complete pathways to disease, and it is then pointless to indict one to the exclusion of the other. The fairest thing to say in such situations is that *either pathway caused the disease*. One sometimes hears it said in such a case that they *both* caused the disease, but this phrase is subject to misinterpretation, that they were each necessary complements of a sufficient cause, which is not what is intended.

There is another problem of causation that is usually described as the direct/indirect dichotomy, but I will argue here that this distinction is actually one of attribution. The basic idea is that we have a *causal chain* $x_2 \longrightarrow x_1 \longrightarrow y$ $[\mathbf{F}]$. Here x_2 is a cause of x_1, and x_1 is a cause of y. This does not imply, of course, that x_2 is a cause of y, but when this does in fact happen, then we say that x_2 is an *indirect cause* acting through x_1, and that x_1 is an *intermediate cause*.

Let us first focus on the consequences of x_1 being an intermediate cause. I want to look at this more generally than I did above, by considering all ways that x_1 might be caused by factors in $\mathbf{F}_1$. There are two ways of considering this. First, I might focus on $C[x_1|\mathbf{F}_1]$, the causes of x_1 generated by $\mathbf{F}_1$. Then $b_1 C[x_1|\mathbf{F}_1]$ consists of pathways in which x_1 was a cause of y, but only through pathways in which x_1 was caused by other elements of $\mathbf{F}$. The other way is to consider $C[b_1 x_1|\mathbf{F}_1]$, which consists of pathways through which other elements of $\mathbf{F}$ cause $b_1 x_1$, which is of course the sufficient causes that contain x_1 as a necessary component. If we had the situation of the preceding paragraph, then the causal equation linking x_2 to x_1 would be a part of these latter two pathways.

Here is part of the argument that pathways in which x_1 is an intermediate cause are ambiguous:

$$b_1 C[x_1|\mathbf{F}_1] \leq b_{0.1} b_1 x_1$$

$$C[b_1 x_1|\mathbf{F}_1] \leq b_{0.1} b_1 x_1$$

To show the top line, first $C[x_1|\mathbf{F}_1] \leq x_1$, so the left side is $\leq b_1 x_1$, and then $b_1 C[x_1|\mathbf{F}_1] \leq b_1 x_1 \xrightarrow{\ s\ } y$ gives $b_1 C[x_1|\mathbf{F}_1] \leq b_{0.1}$. To show the bottom line, $C[b_1 x_1|\mathbf{F}_1] \xrightarrow{\ s\ } C[y|\mathbf{F}_1] = b_{0.1}$, and $C[b_1 x_1|\mathbf{F}_1] \xrightarrow{\ s\ } b_1 x_1$ so that $C[b_1 x_1|\mathbf{F}_1] \leq b_1 x_1$.

No matter which definition we use, all of the occurrences in which some other factor causes x_1 (which then goes on to cause y) are contained in the ambiguous cases with respect to x_1. This shows that if we were to eliminate the attributional ambiguity, either as part of the definition of cause, or as a condition on a variable in a causal system, then we would be ruling out the possibility of causal intermediates. In other words, if by definition or by condition we say that $b_{0.1}b_1x_1 = 0$, then this in effect requires that x_1 be completely exogenous with respect to F_1, in the sense that all of its causes lie outside the descriptive ability possible with F_1. Intermediateness implies attributional ambiguity.

In the opposite situation we have $x_1 \longrightarrow x_2 \longrightarrow y$ [F], and I now turn to this case. Here, we usually say that x_1 is an *indirect cause*, but a more precise statement would be that x_1 acts indirectly through the above causal chain. The reason for this fussiness is that in the MSC approach it is possible (indeed, likely) that a cause will be both direct and indirect, so that these two adjectives are more appropriately applied to causal chains than to factors.

The puzzle is to figure out where the elements of this indirect causal chain reside. First, remember that we have

$$C[y|F] = b_{0.12} \vee b_{1.2}x_1 \vee b_{2.1}x_2 \vee b_{12}x_1x_2 \quad \text{causal}[F]$$

We assume $x_1 \longrightarrow x_2$ [F_2], which means that we also have

$$a_{0.1} \vee a_1x_1 \dashrightarrow x_2 \quad \text{causal}[F_2]$$

Now we might take $b_2a_1x_1$ to consist of all pathways through which x_1 causes x_2 which causes y. First, we have $a_1x_1 \leq C[x_2|F_2]$ so that $b_2a_1x_1 \leq b_{0.2}b_2x_2$, from the results of the first part of this section. Secondly, recall $b_2 = b_{2.1} \vee b_{12}x_1$, so that

$$b_2a_1x_1 = b_{2.1}a_1x_1 \vee b_{12}a_1x_1$$

The second part of this disjunction is a little hard to understand as an instance in which x_1 causes x_2 which causes y, because this latter term is equal to $b_{12}a_1x_1x_2$ which consists of causes that actually involve the joint x_1x_2 pathways. In other words, including these joint causal pathways as part of an indirect causal chain seems to strain the intended notion.

Thus, we might do better to say that $b_{2.1}a_1x_1$ really represents all of the indirect causal chains, from x_1 through x_2 to y. This gives us $b_{2.1}a_1x_1 \leq b_{2.1}x_2 \leq b_{0.1}$. Thus we have

$$b_{2.1}a_1x_1 \leq b_{0.2}b_2x_2b_{0.1}x_1 \leq b_{0.1}x_1$$

This shows that all of the causal chains through which x_1 operates indirectly lie in $b_{0.1}x_1$. It is perhaps worthwhile to note that if we had said that x_1 acts indirectly through x_2 meant $x_1 \longrightarrow b_{2.1}x_2$ [F_2], then we would again have the result that all such causal chains were in $b_{0.1}x_1$.

These considerations motivate the following definition:

$$b_1^i = \vee \{f \in \Pi F_1 : fx_1 \overset{s}{\longrightarrow} b_{0.1}, f \overset{s}{\longmapsto} b_{0.1}\}$$

We call b_1^i the *indirect co-cause* of x_1. This is justified by the causal equation

$$b_{0.1} = b_{0.1} \vee b_1^i x_1 \qquad \text{causal}[F]$$

We thus have

$$b_1^i x_1 \overset{s}{\longrightarrow} b_{0.1} \overset{s}{\longrightarrow} y \quad [F]$$

so that x_1 acts indirectly in this causal chain. We have seen that every pathway through which x_1 acts indirectly in a causal chain is contained in $b_{0.1}$, and so the above is, in a sense, the largest causal chain in which x_1 acts indirectly.

Note that the causal equation for $b_{0.1}$ is occult, in the sense that

$$b_1^i x_1 \leq b_{0.1}$$

so that the causal equation is mathematically equivalent to the tautology $b_{0.1} = b_{0.1}$. This is another case where we have to remember that the purpose of a causal equation (or relation) is to display the minimal sufficient causes, not to capture a mathematical equality. The fact that $b_1^i x_1$ cannot be detected in the causal equation is irrelevant. Its importance stems from its interpretation as the largest collection of indirect causal pathways involving x_1.

The definition that is complementary to the indirect co-cause is the *direct co-cause*

$$b_1^d = \vee \{f \in \Pi F_1 : fx_1 \overset{s}{\longrightarrow} y, fx_1 \overset{s}{\longmapsto} b_{0.1}\}$$

The name is justified, because for f and g in ΠF_1

$$fx_1 \overset{s}{\longrightarrow} g \overset{s}{\longrightarrow} y \Rightarrow fx_1 \overset{s}{\longrightarrow} b_{0.1}$$

104

so that every pathway fx_1 in which x_1 acts indirectly is not part of the definition of $b_1^d x_1$. In particular, we cannot have

$$b_1^d x_1 \dashrightarrow g \dashrightarrow y \qquad \text{(cannot happen)}$$

It is obvious just by looking at the definitions that no f can be in the definitions of both the indirect co-cause and direct co-cause. When we look at the definition of the indirect co-cause, we see that $f \mapsto b_{0.1}$ is equivalent to $f \mapsto y$, and so no harm would be done by (redundantly) adding this latter condition to the definition. By the same token, since $f \dashrightarrow y \Rightarrow fx_1 \dashrightarrow b_{0.1}$, we could also add the (redundant) condition $f \mapsto y$ to the definition of the direct co-cause. But it is then apparent that every f in the definition of b_1 is either in the definition of the indirect co-cause or in the definition of the direct co-cause. In other words, the direct and indirect co-causes partition the pathways of the co-cause. This immediately gives

$$b_1 = b_1^i \vee b_1^d$$

It is now a direct consequence of $b_1^i x_1 \leq b_{0.1}$ that

$$C[y|\mathbf{F}] = b_{0.1} \vee b_1^d x_1$$

This shows that we could have taken the path that led only to direct causal equations, a name that seems to pertain naturally to the above equation, but if we had done that then we would have had some difficulty accounting for indirect causal chains. Having followed the path we did, we can now recognize that it would not be unusual for a cause to have both a nontrivial indirect co-cause and a nontrivial direct co-cause, both at the same time. This would reflect the common-sense notion that it acted directly along some pathways, and indirectly along others. This in turn reinforces the idea that "direct" and "indirect" are properties of causal pathways, not properties of causes themselves.

This has some fairly profound consequences for attempts to define causation by talking about direct and indirect causes, as if that partitioned the collection of causes. It suggests that at some point any such account will come into fairly direct conflict with the minimal sufficient cause principle, although it is perhaps somewhat murky just where that conflict will happen.

Indirect Cause: Probabilities

In this section I want to consider a situation that would usually be described by saying that x_3 causes x_2 which then goes on to cause x_1. In the preceding section I have dealt with some of the complexities of what this means, and so in this section I want to take a simpler view. I assume that the causal diagram of Figure 1 shows all of the relevant causal relationships, and that the IFR holds, so that none of the parameters shown in this figure are miss-specified. This is rather a lot of assumption, but perhaps one of the lessons of preceding chapters is that if we shrink from making any assumptions then we are likely to succumb to analysis paralysis.

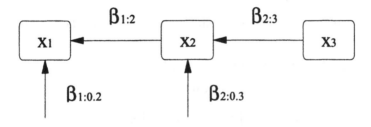

Figure 1. The simple indirect causal diagram.

The question is, given this arrangement what is the causal model relating x_1 to x_3? The first step toward a solution is to accept that the causal diagram shows all the relationships there are. In particular, there is no direct causal pathway from x_3 to x_1, nor is there a joint causal pathway involving x_2 and x_3 as causes of x_1. One of the important points about causal diagrams is that when they leave arrows out, the intention is usually to make the positive assertion that the arrows are not there.

With this convention in mind, Figure 1 can be taken to mean that the only ways in which x_3 can cause x_1 is by first causing x_2. Because of the lack of x_3 to x_1 or $x_2 x_3$ to x_1 pathways, we can write

$$P[x_1=1|x_2,x_3] = \beta_{1:0.2} \vee \beta_{1:2} x_2$$

This implies that $x_1 \amalg x_3 \mid x_2$. Some approaches to causation take this to be the definition that x_3 is an indirect cause of x_1, which in this case acts entirely through x_2. In the next Section we will see how this can fail, but for the moment I assume that this is not a problem.

Now imagine that we were to drop x_2 from F, but that the IFR still held in the causal relation

$$b_{1:03} \vee b_{1:3} x_3 \;\overset{\text{\tiny ■}}{\longrightarrow}\; x_1 \;\; [F_2]$$

so that we would have the correctly specified model

$$P[x_1=1|x_3] = \beta_{1:03} \vee \beta_{1:3} x_3$$

The whole point of this section is to compute these coefficients in terms of those given in Figure 1.

I have introduced the method in Section 16. Here is how it plays out in this situation:

$$P[x_1=1|x_3] = P[x_1=1|x_2=0,x_3]P[x_2=0|x_3]$$
$$+ P[x_1=1|x_2=1,x_3]P[x_2=1|x_3] =$$
$$= \beta_{1:0.2}(\beta_{2:0.3} \vee \beta_{2:3} x_3)^* + (\beta_{1:0.2} \vee \beta_{1:2})(\beta_{2:0.3} \vee \beta_{2:3} x_3)$$
$$= \beta_{1:0.2} \vee \beta_{1:2}(\beta_{2:0.3} \vee \beta_{2:3} x_3)$$
$$= (\beta_{1:0.2} \vee \beta_{1:2}\beta_{2:0.3}) \vee (\beta_{1:2} \backslash \beta_{1:2}\beta_{2:0.3})\beta_{2:3} x_3$$

In other words,

$$\beta_{1:0.3} = \beta_{1:0.2} \vee \beta_{1:2}\beta_{2:0.3}$$

$$\beta_{1:3} = (\beta_{1:2} \backslash \beta_{1:2}\beta_{2:03})\beta_{2:3}$$

These equations show how to transform the two direct causal relationships in Figure 1 into the single direct causal relationship that results from dropping x_2. Note that the first equation above can be interpreted as the residual pathways into x_1 together with the residuals into

x_2 which then have their effect on x_1. The second equation is interesting because we might have imagined that it would turn out to be $\beta_{1:2}\beta_{2:3}$. In order to understand this, it is helpful to pose the structural causal models

$$x_1 = b_{1:0.2} \vee b_{1:2} x_2$$

$$x_2 = b_{2:0.3} \vee b_{2:3} x_3$$

so that by direct substitution and simplification

$$x_1 = b_{1:0.2} \vee b_{1:2}(b_{2:0.3} \vee b_{2:3} x_3) = (b_{1:0.2} \vee b_{1:2} b_{2:0.3}) \vee b_{1:2} b_{2:3} x_3$$

I have made no argument that the term in parentheses on the right is the residual, nor that the coefficient of x_3 is the co-cause, but the point here is that in moving from this structural model to the probability model, the considerations that arise are similar to what we have seen before. In particular, we cannot have the coefficient of x_3 independent of the term in parentheses, and this is what prevents the probability model from having $\beta_{1:2}\beta_{2:3}$ as the coefficient of x_3. We might refer to this phenomenon as *intrinsic miss-specification*, and observe that it will happen often when we deal with indirect causes.

Table 1 provides some data illustrating simple indirect causation. This study is an example of a type that has become more and more prevalent in the latter half of this century, in which one does not investigate some scientific issue, but instead studies other studies. Of course, causal analysis has just as much place in methodology studies as it does in proper scientific studies.

Type of arthritis	Comparison	Dropped Out
Osteo	Placebo	18/552 = 0.033
	Other drug	17/585 = 0.029
Rheumatoid	Placebo	126/844 = 0.149
	Other drug	165/1252 = 0.132

Journal of Clinical Epidemiology 1999;52(2):113-122

Table 1. Results from a study of studies of NSAID treatment of arthritis. Dropped-out indicates participants who quit the trial because they felt their therapy was ineffective.

The idea behind the methodology study was that whether or not the scientific study used a placebo control might influence the outcome. Rather than look at the actual treatment outcomes, the authors looked at indicators of the conduct of the trial, and in particular the number of individuals who dropped out because they felt they were being given an ineffective therapy. It is plausible that if they knew that one of the therapies was a placebo (and so they had a 50-50 chance of getting it) they might have less patience than if they felt they were getting some drug regardless of which treatment group they fell into.

Let us take d = dropped out, c = drug comparison, and r = rheumatoid arthritis. We can then easily compute the path coefficients for Figure 2. The conclusion is obviously that the type of arthritis (r) causes dropping out, but that there are no pathways involving either the design (c) or joint pathways involving both factors. It is also apparent that the design (c) causes the type of arthritis studies (r). Note that it is biologically plausible that rheumatoid arthritis would cause more drop-outs than osteoarthritis would. It may seem strange, however, to say that having a drug comparison causes the study to be of rheumatoid arthritis. What this points up is that there can be different kinds of causation acting in the same setting. The first kind may be biological, and the second kind may mean that investigators who chose drug comparisons tended to *select* to study rheumatoid arthritis. As many scientists learn to their chagrin, selection can be a very potent causal force in biomedical experiments.

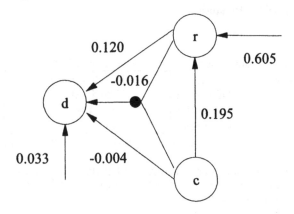

Figure 2. Causal diagram for the data in Table 1.

We are, therefore, justified in depicting the situation as in Figure 3. The path coefficients can be computed simply from the data in Table 1. Applying the formulas derived in this section (and identifying d with x_1 and c with x_3):

$$\beta_{1:0.3} = 0.031 \vee (0.111)(0.605) = 0.096$$

$$\beta_{1:3} = (0.111 \setminus (0.111)(0.605))0.195 = 0.009$$

We would conclude that although c may be an indirect cause of d, unless one of the specification assumptions has failed, it is a very weak cause.

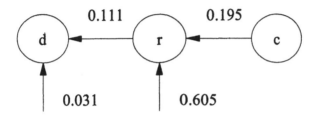

Figure 3. Causal diagram showing c acting indirectly through r.

We would usually expect the situation to be what it was here, where we needed to fit a more elaborate model, and then prune out the practically insignificant paths, ending up with an indirect cause model. In some other, perhaps less frequent cases, we might be able to stipulate an indirect cause model out of the logic of the observations themselves. A leading example of this type would be when x_3 is randomization to treatment x_2, and the treatment causes recovery from disease x_1. Since we do not have all the pieces yet that we will need for this case, I postpone it to Section 28.

Indirect Cause: Structures

In the preceding Section I looked at indirect causation from a simple point of view. The relationships there are the ones that we would want to hold to give a coherent meaning to the concept of indirect cause. Unfortunately the world does not always cater to our whims, and the purpose of this section is to see what might go wrong.

Throughout this section I assume that x_1 is a cause of y only because x_1 is a cause of x_2 and x_2 then goes on to cause y. This leads me to posit the causal equation

$$C[x_2|F] = b_{2:0.1} \vee b_{2:1}x_1 \qquad causal[F_2]$$

and the inequality

$$b_1x_1 \le b_{2.1}b_{2:1}x_1$$

The causal equation simply establishes that x_1 is a cause of x_2, but the inequality says that all pathways in which x_1 is a cause of y can be seen as cases in which x_1 caused x_2, and then x_2 went on to cause y.

From the results of Section 14, the inequality and causal equation imply

$$b_{1.2}x_1 \vee b_{12}x_1x_2 \le b_{2.1}x_2$$

This immediately gives

$$C[y|F] = b_{0.12} \vee b_{2.1}x_2$$

There are several reasons why this is a very satisfying equation, but also one that is difficult to understand. First, it is not a causal equation. Recall that the purpose of a causal equation is to list all of the minimal sufficient causes, usually from the perspective that some factors are measured and many others are not. Thus, the causal equation is still

$$C[y|F] = b_{0.12} \vee b_{1.2}x_1 \vee b_{2.1}x_2 \vee b_{12}x_1x_2 \qquad causal[F]$$

and the fact that some of the terms in this expression are dominated by others is of mathematical importance, but not necessarily of causal importance.

Secondly, in the equation

$$C[y|\mathbf{F}] = b_{0.12} \vee b_{2.1}x_2$$

the right side is in $\vee\Pi\mathbf{F}_1$, and this immediately implies

$$C[y|\mathbf{F}_1] = b_{0.12} \vee b_{2.1}x_2 \qquad \text{causal}[\mathbf{F}_1]$$

This underscores once again that there is a difference between mathematical and causal equations, and that the selection of the causal field is part of what distinguishes the two.

My immediate objective is to compute $P[y{=}1|x_1,x_2]$ under the assumptions I have made above, and the preceding equation is the key. Again to ease the notation I temporarily assume that $y = C[y|\mathbf{F}]$.

First compute

$$P[y{=}1|x_1,x_2{=}0] = P[b_{0.12}{=}1|x_1,x_2{=}0] = \beta_{0.12} \vee \delta_{0.1.2}x_1$$

Then compute

$$P[y{=}1|x_1,x_2{=}1] = P[b_{0.12}{=}1|x_1,x_2{=}1]\vee P[b_{2.1}{=}1|x_1,x_2{=}1,b_{0.12}{=}0]$$

$$= \beta_{0.12} \vee \delta_{0.1.2}x_1 \vee \delta_{0.2.1} \vee \delta_{0.12}x_1 \vee \beta_{2.1} \vee \delta_{1.2}x_1$$

Consequently,

$$P[y{=}1|x_1,x_2] = \beta_{0.12} \vee \delta_{0.1.2}x_1 \vee (\beta_{2.1}\vee\delta_{0.2.1})x_2 \vee (\delta_{0.12}\vee\delta_{1.2})x_1x_2$$

This equation has been derived just from the assumption that x_1 causes y only through its effect on x_2. An exceedingly natural way to express this condition in probability terms is

$$y \perp\!\!\!\perp x_1 \mid x_2$$

This says that once one fixes x_2 (however that might be done), there is no probability relationship between y and x_1. Another way of saying the same thing is

$$P[y{=}1|x_1,x_2] = P[y{=}1|x_2]$$

Now go back one paragraph to see that the expression I derived, assuming x_1 caused y only through x_2, is not of this form. It depends not only on x_2, but also on x_1 and x_1x_2.

114

What is wrong here? The most obvious fact is that all of the parameters that keep y from being conditionally independent of x_1 given x_2 are δ-parameters. That is, they all come from one of the model misspecification sources that I identified in Section 12. If we assume IFR then we get

$$P[y=1|x_1,x_2] = \beta_{0.12} \vee \beta_{2.1}x_2 \vee \delta_{1.2}x_1x_2$$

This is not enough to free y from x_1. We must also assume half of CIFC in order to achieve the desired equation

$$P[y=1|x_1,x_2] = \beta_{0.12} \vee \beta_{2.1}x_2$$

These results have some practical and philosophical consequences. One philosophical implication is that any attempt to define indirect causation in terms of probability models is going to have to make a prior assumption that the models are, in an appropriate sense, correctly causally specified. We have just seen that if either IFR or the relevant half of CIFC fail, then conditional independence will not serve as a definition of indirect causation. Thus, the definition of Suppes[1] and its later, very considerable extension by Spirtes, Glymour, and Scheines[2] appears to rest on a rather strong assumption about model specification. The same comment applies to the more restricted classical linear "causal" models, which constitute most of the currently received wisdom about causal analysis throughout social science.

The practical implication follows from the philosophical consequences. One cannot simply fit causal models (however defined) and conclude that when x_2 remains in the model but x_1 falls out (due to statistical significance considerations) that x_1 can be at best an indirect cause. The additional assumptions necessary for this have to do with correct specification of the causal field, and correct specification of the model within the causal field. If there are errors in these specifications, then the naïve statistical inference may fail.

In more general terms, these considerations lead back to one of the dominant themes of this book. Our ability to study a causal system is better to the extent that we have measured the important causal factors, and analyzed our data using causal models that employ these factors in an explanatory role. It is probably true that no matter how far we go down this path, we will never be sure that unwanted associations might make some (or all) of our causal parameters mis-specified. But measuring more (rather than less), and analyzing more (rather than less) is the only rational attack on this problem.

References

1. Suppes P. A probabilistic theory of causality. Acta Philosophica Fennica Fasc. XXIV. Amsterdam, The Netherlands: North-Holland Publishing Company, 1970
2. Spirtes P, Glymour C, Scheines R. Causation, Prediction, and Search. Lecture Notes in Statistics 81. New York NY: Springer-Verlag. 1993

20

Reversal

The Reversal Equations. If we assume the causal relation

$$b_{1:0.2} \vee b_{1:2}x_2 \; \overset{\textbf{s}}{\dashrightarrow} \; x_1 \quad [\textbf{F}]$$

and the IFR, then we have

$$P[x_1=1|x_2] = \beta_{1:0.2} \vee \beta_{1:2}x_2$$

From the fundamental definition of conditional probability, we have

$$P\big[x_2 = j\big|x_1 = i\big] = P\big[x_1 = i\big|x_2 = j\big]\frac{P\big[x_2 = j\big]}{P\big[x_1 = i\big]}$$

This equation is often called "Bayes' Theorem", which is an historical oddity, since the Thomas Bayes who unwittingly donated his name to this equation barely had anything like the modern concept of probability in mind. In fact, the equation is just another way to express the definition of conditional probability, so it is a tautology, Bayes' Tautology.

It is clear that from this that I can state

$$P[x_2=1|x_1] = \beta_{2:0.1} \vee \beta_{2:1}x_1$$

and that Bayes' Tautology should connect $\beta_{2:0.1}$ and $\beta_{2:1}$ with $\beta_{1:0.2}$ and $\beta_{1:2}$. In fact, to complete the story we need to define

$$P[x_1=1] = \xi_1$$

$$P[x_2=1] = \xi_2$$

Here are the *reversal equations* that relate all these parameters:

(1) $\xi_1 = \beta_{1:0.2} \vee \beta_{1:2}\xi_2$

(2) $\xi_2 = \beta_{2:0.1} \vee \beta_{2:1}\xi_1$

(3) $\beta_{2:0.1}*\xi_1* = \beta_{1:0.2}*\xi_2*$

(4) $\beta_{2:1}\xi_1 = \beta_{1:2}\xi_2$

To derive these equations, first note that (1) and (2) are examples of computations I have given before. Equation (3) is an instance of Bayes' Tautology

$$\beta_{2:0.1}* = P[x_2=0|x_1=0] = P[x_1=0|x_2=0]P[x_2=0]/P[x_1=0] =$$

$$= \beta_{1:0.2}*\xi_2*/\xi_1*$$

To get (4), again start with Bayes' Tautology in the form

$$(\beta_{2:0.1}\vee\beta_{2:1})\xi_1 = (\beta_{1:0.2}\vee\beta_{1:2})\xi_2$$

and re-express it as

$$\beta_{2:1}\xi_1 \vee (\xi_1\backslash\xi_1\beta_{2:1})\beta_{2:0.1} = \beta_{1:2}\xi_2 \vee (\xi_2\backslash\xi_2\beta_{2:1})\beta_{1:0.2}$$

Now I claim that $\beta_{1.0.2} = \xi_1\backslash\xi_1\beta_{2:1}$ and that $\beta_{2:0.1} = \xi_2\backslash\xi_2\beta_{2:1}$, which will clearly give (4). By the symmetry in the notation, I only have to establish the first of these latter claims. This comes from the following lines:

$\beta_{1:0.2}*\xi_2* = \beta_{2:0.1}*\xi_1*$ (which is (3))

$\beta_{1:0.2} \vee \xi_2 = \beta_{2:0.1} \vee \xi_1$

$\beta_{1:0.2} \vee \beta_{2:0.1} \vee \beta_{2:1}\xi_1 = \beta_{2:0.1} \vee \xi_1$ (from (2))

$\beta_{1:0.2} = \xi_1\backslash\xi_1\beta_{2:1}$

This completes the demonstration of the reversal equations.

It is worth noting how many parameters there really are here. There are altogether four β-parameters and two ξ-parameters, for a total of six parameters. There are then the four reversal equations that connect these parameters; however, any one of the reversal equations can be deduced from the other three, so there are really only three independent equations. And consequently there are really only three independent parameters (six nominal parameters minus three equations). Which three one regards as basic depends on one's point of view, or what evidence one has. The important thing here is that one can specify any three of the parameters, and then obtain the remainder by clever use of the reversal equations.

Surrogate Measures. Perhaps the leading example of this kind of situation concerns a so-called *surrogate*. There are other terms for this, such as *marker*, but this latter name is used in so many different contexts without adequate definition that I will stick with *surrogate*. The basic idea is displayed in Figure 1. Here, x_1 is a factor that we want to measure, but for some reason we can't. We can, however, measure another factor, the surrogate x_2, of which x_1 is a cause. Note that Figure 1 explicitly defines three of the parameters that link x_1 and x_2.

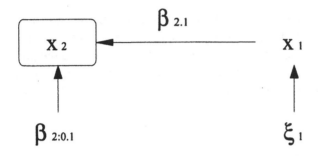

Figure 1. A surrogate (x_2) is caused by an unmeasured factor (x_1).

As a concrete example, let x_1 be gestational diabetes mellitus (GDM). This is a disease that strikes pregnant women, and which has the same form as diabetes - inability to move glucose (sugar) from the bloodstream into the cells where it is needed. Unlike diabetes, GDM usually disappears after delivery, although women who have had GDM in one pregnancy frequently have it again in subsequent pregnancies, and have an increased chance of eventually becoming diabetics. The condition must be treated during pregnancy to prevent severe problems with the baby.

GDM is a disease, and we cannot directly measure whether the disease entity "diabetes" is present in any given woman. The best we can do is to perform a clinical test, and on the basis of the test to diagnose the woman as GDM or not. The usual test administers 50 grams of oral glucose to the woman and then measures her concentration of plasma glucose one hour later; a value greater than 140 milligrams per deciliter constitutes a GDM diagnosis.

In this case, the diagnosis is the surrogate for the disease. The reason for this is that the disease is the impairment of the system which moves glucose into cells, but the test does not measure this impairment directly. Instead it measures something that is caused by the impairment, too much glucose left in the blood. Another reason to take this view is that if we perform the test several times over a period of weeks, we may find different test results. It does not make much sense to imagine that the woman shifts back and forth between GDM and health; a better explanation is that there are other things that act as causes of the test result.

In the diagnostic test example it is a convention to specify the *sensitivity* of the test, which is the probability of a positive test in someone who has the disease, and the *specificity* of the test, which is the probability of a negative test in someone who does not have the disease. Converting these to causal parameters (with x_2 as the test and x_1 as the disease) we have

$$\text{sensitivity} = \beta_{2:0.1} \vee \beta_{2:1}$$

$$\text{specificity} = \beta_{2:0.1}{}^*$$

so that

$$\beta_{2:1} = \text{sensitivity} \setminus \text{specificity*}$$

Although the sensitivity/specificity designation is a little awkward from the causal perspective, we have to remember that these terms were codified in an era when the appreciation of the importance of causal quantification was weaker than it is today.

For GDM in the United States, the accepted figures are[1] sensitivity = 0.83, specificity = 0.87. Consequently,

$$\beta_{2:0.1} = 0.13$$

$$\beta_{2:1} = 0.83 \setminus 0.13 = .80$$

The final element of the troika of parameters is the probability of disease for a woman randomly sampled from pregnancies (the *prevalence* of GDM), which is again accepted[1] to be about 0.03, so that

$$\xi_1 = 0.03$$

This situation is summarized in the causal diagram of Figure 2.

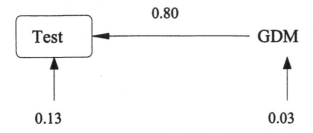

Figure 2. The classical diagnostic test causal diagram, here for a glucose tolerance test as a surrogate for gestational diabetes (GDM)

We apply the reversal equations as follows. First,

$$\xi_2 = \beta_{2:0.1} \vee \beta_{2:1}\xi_1 = 0.13 \vee (0.80)(0.03) = 0.15$$

which is the prevalence of positive GDM tests (if they were given to everyone, or a random sample of everyone). The next steps are

$$\beta_{1:0.2} = (\beta_{2:0.1}{}^*\xi_1{}^*/\xi_2{}^*)^* = ((0.13)^*(0.03)^*/(0.15)^*)^* =$$
$$= ((0.87)(0.97)/0.85)^* = 0.01$$
$$\beta_{1:2} = \beta_{2:1}\xi_1/\xi_2 = (0.80)(0.03)/0.15 = 0.16$$

These results are shown in Figure 3. Note here that the arrow connecting x_1 to x_2 does not correspond to a causal relation, because the GDM test is not a cause of the disease. Reversal is a process that reverses conditional probability distributions, which may or may not represent a reversal of the causal process. In this case, it does not.

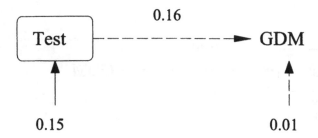

Figure 3. Reversal of Figure 2. The arrows pointing to GDM represent probability relationships, that may not be causal.

The parameters in Figure 3 are usually used in the following fashion. If a woman has a negative test, then conditional on this her probability of having GDM is 0.01. If her test is positive, then conditional on this her probability of having GDM is $0.01 \vee 0.16 = 0.17$. The latter is usually called the *positive predictive probability (PPP)* while the $0.01^* = 0.99$ is the *negative predictive probability (NPP)*. These are awkward terms, and have been slightly reformulated into other, equally awkward terms in various disciplines where diagnostic tests are used.

From the viewpoint of this section, the important fact is that it is possible to go from the situation in Figure 2 to that in Figure 3 without any computational difficulty. The reversal equations are fundamental to this process, because they show how reversal impacts causal parameters.

Reference

1. Singer DE. Samet JH, Coley CM, Nathan DM. Screening for diabetes mellitus. In Eddy DM (ed.) Common Screening Tests. Philadelphia PA: American College of Physicians. 1991, Ch..6

Gestational Diabetes Example

In the preceding Section we saw how the reversal equations permitted us to convert the causal effect of a disease on a test into a probability relationship between a test and the disease. This fact has some considerable impact on the assessment of the causal effects of the disease, which is often ignored.

Returning to the GDM example, the main immediate problems caused by the disease are complications with the baby. Let us use y for such a complication, x_2 for the oral glucose test for GDM, and x_1 for GDM itself. We typically start with the situation in Figure 1, where we have some data relating the occurrence of a positive test (x_2) with subsequent occurrence of the complication (y). In this figure, the causal parameters connecting x_1 with x_2 are those that we derived in the preceding section. The $\beta_{0.2}$ and β_2 parameters are not causal, but only probability parameters expressed in the causal form using unitary algebra. Since these parameters relate y to the surrogate x_2, we could call them *surrogate effects*.

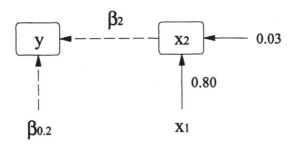

Figure 1. Diagram for a study of surrogate effects.

The actual causal situation is shown in Figure 2. The complication (y) is caused by the disease (x_1), and the test (x_2) is also caused by the disease. There is no arrow connecting x_2 with y because in a causal field that includes x_1, x_2 has no causal effect on y. The central question is, how do we get from the information in Figure 1 to the values of the causal parameters $\beta_{0.12}$ and $\beta_{1.2}$ in Figure 2?

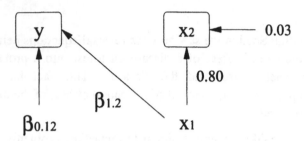

Figure 2. Causal diagram corresponding to Figure 1.

The first part of the answer is to reverse the causal connection from x_1 to x_2 in Figure 2. This was done in the preceding Section, and is shown here in Figure 3. But now we can see that Figure 3 is identical to Figure 1 of Section 18. In that figure the arrows were all causal, whereas here two of the arrows are probabilistic, but insofar as the computations of model parameters are concerned, this is irrelevant.

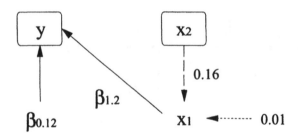

Figure 3. Diagram obtained from Figure 2 by reversal.

Thus we have the equation

$$\beta_{0.2} \vee \beta_2 x_2 = \beta_{0.12} \vee \beta_{1.2}(0.01 \vee 0.16 x_2)$$

which implies

$$\beta_{0.2} = \beta_{0.12} \vee 0.01\beta_{1.2}$$

$$\beta_2 = (\beta_{1.2} \setminus 0.01\beta_{1.2})(0.16)$$

The solutions of these equations are

$$\beta_{1.2} = \beta_2/((0.99)(0.16) + (0.01)\beta_2) = \beta_2/(0.158+0.01\beta_2)$$

$$\beta_{0.12} = \beta_{0.2} \setminus \beta_{1.2}$$

These equations show how to convert an "observed" relationship between the test and the complication to the actual underlying causal relationship between the disease and the complication. Perhaps the most important point is that $\beta_{1.2}$ will always exceed β_2. In other words, if we accept "test-complication" association as the measure of "disease-complication" effect, we will underestimate the latter.

Since we have, in effect, built a small engine for converting observed effects to causal effects in the GDM situation, let us now apply it to some examples.

Probability of Congenital Malformation	
GDM	248/8869 = 0.028
Non-GDM	188/8934 = 0.021

Paediatric Perinatal Epidemiology 1996;10(1):52-63

Table 1. Chance of a congenital malformation for GDM and non-GDM births.

In Table 1 we have $\beta_2 = 0.028 \setminus 0.021 = 0.0072$, indicating an effect of a little more than 7 per thousand births. Converting to the causal effect, $\beta_{1.2} = 0.0072/(0.158 +0.000072) = 0.0454$, which is about 45 per thousand births. This is a rather important result. Even though the oral glucose test for GDM is regarded as being reasonably good (sensitivity = 0.83, specificity = 0.87), relying on the test to establish the causal effect of GDM on congenital malformations understates the actual causal effect by a factor of six. A critical issue here is that the GDM women who participated in this study were certainly treated for their condition, since it would unethical to permit them to suffer the higher occurrence of birth complications that is known to follow from GDM, simply to estimate how much higher it is. Therefore, the actual disease here is "treated GDM", and it is easy to see that one might prefer the 7/1000 congenital malformation probability to the 45/1000 probability, if one wanted to make the argument that the treatment was effective. A causal analysis suggests that either the treatment is not as effective as it appears, or else there are other characteristics of GDM women that cause them to produce malformed infants even when their blood sugar is therapeutically controlled. Which (if any) of these scenarios is correct would the subject of another study.

Table 2 shows some additional examples of the probability of unwanted consequences among GDM and Non-GDM mothers. Notice that in the case of macrosomia (child with large body) 82% of treated GDM women who have escaped the residual causes of this complication would experience it nonetheless. This is a large causal effect, which is seriously understated by the β_2 estimates based on the test alone.

Complication	GDM	Non-GDM	β_2	$\beta_{1:2}$
Macrosomia	0.179	0.056	0.130	0.816
Polycythemia	0.133	0.049	0.088	0.554
Hyperbilirubinemia	0.165	0.082	0.090	0.566
Hypocalcemia	0.035	0.027	0.008	0.051

Diabetes Care 1998;21(supp 2)::B79-B84

Table 2. Several birth complication probabilities among GDM and Non-GDM women

The lesson of these examples is clear. When estimation of a causal effect is based on a surrogate factor, rather than on the actual factor itself, then one may expect to see smaller effects, and sometimes much smaller effects. Conversely, reports that do not convert to correct causal effects systematically understate the magnitude of those causal effects. These facts are not widely appreciated in the biomedical community, which has resulted in a ubiquitous distortion in the scientific literature.

One must be careful to keep in mind, however, that these results rest on the assumption that the models are correctly specified. We should be aware by now that there is always a hoard of disagreeable possibilities lurking in the background, any one of which is capable of leading us astray.

More Reversal

In this section I would like to consolidate the material of the two preceding sections. The causal situation is shown on the left side in Figure 1. The relationship I am interested in is the causal $x_1 \longrightarrow x_2$ [F]. There are two problems. First, as shown in the figure, I only have surrogate x_3 for x_1 and surrogate x_4 for x_2. Secondly, in addition to the parameters connecting the factors with their surrogages ($\beta_{3:0.1}, \beta_{3:3}, \beta_{4:0.2}, \beta_{4:2}$) the data I have will only connect the surrogates, to compute $\beta_{4:0.3}$ and $\beta_{4:3}$.

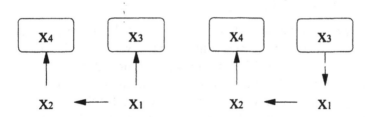

Figure 1. The left side shows the causal model, while the right side shows the situation with one arrow reversed.

The strategy is conceptually simple, to express $\beta_{4:0.3}$ and $\beta_{4:3}$ in terms of the other parameters, giving two equations from which $\beta_{2:0.1}$ and $\beta_{2:1}$ can be obtained. The first step is obviously to reverse the arrow from x_1 to x_3, as shown on the right in Figure 1. How to do this was covered in Section 20.

At this point it is convenient to review how conditional expectation works with unitary algebra. The reason for doing this is that it simplifies some of the computations. First, observe that

$$P[y=1|x_1] = \beta_{0.1} \vee \beta_1 x_1$$

means the same as

$$E[y|x_1] = \beta_{0.1} \vee \beta_1 x_1$$

As an aside, note that this makes it obvious that

$$E[y] = \beta_{0.1} \vee \beta_1 E[x_1]$$

an equation I deduced before, and have used much since. What I want to point out here is the validity of some more complex relationships. For example, suppose that

$$E[y|x_1,x_2] = \beta_{0.12} \vee \beta_{1.2} x_1 \vee \beta_{2.1} x_2 \vee \beta_{12} x_1 x_2$$

Then

$$E[y|x_1] = E[E[y|x_1,x_2]\,|x_1] = \beta_{0.12} \vee \beta_{1.2} x_1 \vee (\beta_{2.1} \vee \beta_{12} x_1) E[x_2|x_1]$$

We now set up the equations required to solve the problem of Figure 1. Start with

$$\beta_{4:0.3} \vee \beta_{4:3} x_3 = E[E[x_4\,|x_1,x_2,x_3]\,|x_3]$$

It is important on the left side of Figure 1 that the absence of arrows directly from x_1 or x_3 to x_4 means that $x_4 \amalg x_1, x_3 \mid x_2$. This means first, that the cause x_1 affects the surrogate x_4 only through its impact on the effect x_2, and secondly, there is no relationship (causal or otherwise) connecting the surrogate x_3 with surrogate x_4, except that created by the fact that they are both caused by the factors x_1 and x_2, which are causally linked. The assumption then justifies

$$E[x_4|x_1,x_2,x_3] = E[x_4|x_2] = \beta_{4:0.2} \vee \beta_{4:2} x_2$$

The preceding equation therefore becomes

$$\beta_{4:0.3} \vee \beta_{4:3} x_3 = \beta_{4:0.2} \vee \beta_{4:2} E[x_2|x_3]$$

Now observe that the absence of a direct arrow from x_3 to x_2 says that $x_3 \amalg x_2 \mid x_1$. Thus

$$E[x_2|x_3] = E[E[x_2|x_1,x_3]|x_3] = E[E[x_2|x_1]|x_3] = \beta_{2:0.1} \vee \beta_{2:1} E[x_1|x_3]$$

The final piece is

$$E[x_1|x_3] = \beta_{1:0.3} \vee \beta_{1:3} x_3$$

Putting these altogether,

$$\beta_{4:0.3} \vee \beta_{4:3} x_3 = \beta_{4:.0.2} \vee \beta_{4:2}(\beta_{2:0.1} \vee \beta_{2:1}(\beta_{1:0.3} \vee \beta_{1:3} x_3))$$

Successively substituting $x_3 = 0,1$ gives two equations

$$\beta_{4:0.3} = \beta_{4:.0.2} \vee \beta_{4:2}(\beta_{2:0.1} \vee \beta_{2:1}\beta_{1:0.3})$$

$$\beta_{4:.0.3} \vee \beta_{4:3} = \beta_{4:.0.2} \vee \beta_{4:2}(\beta_{2:0.1} \vee \beta_{2:1}(\beta_{1:0.3} \vee \beta_{1:3}))$$

The only parameters not known are $\beta_{2:0.1}$ and $\beta_{2:1}$, so that in principle we can solve for them.

Although this looks formidable, with a few preliminary adjustments the problem is easily reduced to the following:

Given a_1, a_2, b_1, b_2, solve $u \vee a_1 v = b_1$, $u \vee a_2 v = b_2$

To solve this, first eliminate u to obtain

$$b_1 \backslash a_1 v = b_2 \backslash a_2 v$$

$$b_1 \backslash b_2 = a_2 v \backslash a_1 v = (a_2 - a_1)v/(a_1 v)^*$$

$$(b_1 \backslash b_2)(a_1 v)^* = (b_1 \backslash b_2) - (b_1 \backslash b_2)a_1 v = (a_2 - a_1)v$$

and so

$$v = (b_1 \backslash b_2)/(a_2 - a_1 + (b_1 \backslash b_2)a_1) = (b_1 - b_2)/(a_2 b_2^* - a_1 b_1^*)$$

Secondly, eliminate v to obtain

$$b_1 \backslash u = (a_1/a_2)(b_2 \backslash u)$$

$$b_1^*/u^* = (a_1/a_2)^* \vee (b_2^*/u^*) = (a_1/a_2)^* + (a_1/a_2)b_2^*/u^*$$

$$b_1^* = (a_1/a_2)^* u^* + (a_1/a_2)b_2^*$$

$$u^* = (b_1^* - (a_1/a_2)b_2^*)/(a_1^* \backslash a_2^*) = (a_2 b_1^* - a_1 b_2^*)/(a_1^* - a_2^*)$$

$$u = (a_1 b_2 - a_2 b_1)/(a_1 - a_2)$$

This solves our little subproblem, and provides a method for obtaining $\beta_{2:0.1}$ and $\beta_{2:1}$ in actual cases.

In principle, this completely solves the problem of reconstructing the actual causal parameters in $x_1 \longrightarrow x_2$ [F] when I must rely on data connecting surrogates in the probability relation $x_3 \longrightarrow x_4$. It is worthwhile remembering, however, what additional information and assumptions I need in order to do this. First, I must have auxiliary studies for the surrogate causal relationships $x_1 \longrightarrow x_3$ [F] and $x_2 \longrightarrow x_4$ [F]. Next, I must assure that the surrogate measures do not have a residual interrelationship, beyond that which is implied by the last two causal relationships. An example where this often fails is when both surrogates are measured at the same time and place, since there are often special circumstances that will influence both of them, independently of their relationships to x_1 and x_2. This is why, for example, one must be wary of questionnaire items that purport to measure exposure to potential causes of disease on the one hand, and the diseases themselves on the other, when both sets of items are on the same form, administered at the same time. Finally, the surrogate x_4 (usually the measure of disease) must not be caused by x_1 by any other pathway than that through the actual disease. For example, if the presence of the x_1 factor influenced how a respondent marked certain items on a questionnaire, independently of whether or not they had the disease, then this latter condition fails.

Since the failure of these conditions simply implies more arrows on the right in Figure 1, we could, in theory, still set up equations and solve for the causal parameters of interest. This would, however, imply that we know a great deal about our surrogate measures, in terms of how they are influenced by various factors. Researchers seldom have this knowledge. In fact, it is customary in most biomedical research to ignore the surrogate issue altogether.

Although it may not be obvious, in Figure 1 the relationship between the surrogates will always be weaker than that between the underlying factors. We can see this easily in two extreme conditions. First, suppose $\beta_{4:0.2}=0$, $\beta_{4:2}=1$. This says that there is no surrogate problem with x_2. The equation to be solved for $\beta_{2:01}$ and $\beta_{2:1}$ is then

$$\beta_{4:03} \vee \beta_{4:3} x_3 = \beta_{2:01} \vee \beta_{2:1}(\beta_{1:03} \vee \beta_{1:3} x_3)$$

We can re-write this in a handy form for our method of solution:

$$\underbrace{\beta_{4:03} \vee \beta_{4:3}}_{b_1} = \beta_{2:01} \vee \beta_{2:1} \underbrace{\left(\beta_{1:03} \vee \beta_{1:3}\right)}_{a_1}$$

$$\underbrace{\beta_{4:03}}_{b_2} = \beta_{2:01} \vee \beta_{2:1} \underbrace{\beta_{1:03}}_{a_2}$$

then

$$\beta_{2:1} = \frac{\beta_{4:03} \vee \beta_{4:3} - \beta_{4:03}}{\beta_{1:03}\beta^{*}_{4:03} - \left(\beta_{1:03} \vee \beta_{1:3}\right)\beta^{*}_{4:03}\beta^{*}_{4:3}} = \frac{\beta_{4:3}}{\beta_{1:03} - \left(\beta_{1:03} \vee \beta_{1:3}\right)\beta^{*}_{4:3}}$$

This shows that $\beta_{2:1}$ will generally exceed $\beta_{4:3}$.

The other extreme situation is $\beta_{1:03}=0$, $\beta_{1:3}=1$, so that there is no surrogate problem with x_1. Here the relevant equation is

$$\beta_{4:03}\vee\beta_{4:3}x_3 = \beta_{4:02}\vee\beta_{4:2}(\beta_{2:01}\vee\beta_{2:1}x_3)$$

from which we can directly compute

$$\beta_{2:1} = \beta_{4:3}/(\beta_{4:2}\backslash\beta_{4:2}\beta_{2:01})$$

so that again $\beta_{2:1}$ exceeds $\beta_{4:3}$. As a reminder, we see these two extreme situations in Figure 2.

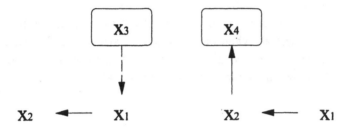

Figure 2. Special cases of Figure 1, in which one factor has no surrogate problem. In both of these cases, the causal relationship $x_1{\rightarrow}x_2$ is stronger than the probability relationships $x_3{\rightarrow}x_2$ or $x_1{\rightarrow}x_4$.

The final example of this section is cautionary. The situation is shown in Figure 3. Up to this point, reversing arrows has been simple, the method having been worked out in Section 20. Figure 3 looks like the same problem, but it is actually harder.

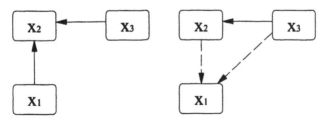

Figure 3. Reversing the diagram on the left gives a diagram of the form on the right.

The problem is the two arrows pointing into x_2. This is the single fact that distinguishes this from earlier examples. The probability principle that one must apply is a version of Bayes' Tautology:

$$pr(x_1|x_2,x_3) = pr(x_2|x_1,x_3)pr(x_1|x_3)/pr(x_2|x_3)$$

This expression simplifies, since the diagram on the left implies that x_1 and x_3 are independent, and moreover by the chain rule

$$pr(x_2|x_3) = \Sigma\ pr(x_2|x_1,x_3)pr(x_1|x_3) = \Sigma\ pr(x_2|x_1,x_3)pr(x_1)$$

(summation over x_1). Nevertheless, even with these simplifications, the expression for $pr(x_1|x_2,x_3)$ still depends on both x_2 and x_3, which accounts for the appearance of the unexpected arrow from x_3 to x_1 on the right side of Figure 3. In general, when one reverses an arrow in a diagram, one must do the reversal conditional on all factors that have arrows pointing into *either* of the two factors involved in the reversal.

Double Reversal

The situation of this section is again one in which I am interested in the causal relation $x_2 \longrightarrow x_1$ [**F**], as shown at the left in Figure 1 below. As in Section 20 when I discussed reversal, I assume I am in the situation where the data at hand permit me to obtain the parameters of the reversed, probability diagram, at the right of Figure 1. The critical issue here is the relationship between the sampling that was done to obtain the data and a random sample from the population of opportunities. Since I have used P for a random draw from Ω, let me use P' to denote the probability under ·which the right side of Figure 1 was obtained.

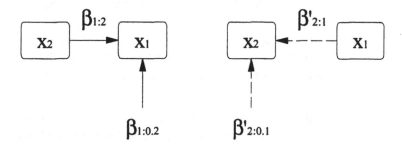

Figure 1. The left side shows the causal situation corresponding to sampling with P, while the right side shows the data available, sampled with P' .

If P = P', then the situation of Section 20 applies, and the reversal procedure given there would work here. In this section I want to extend this to cases where P and P' differ. For convenience in working with distributions, I let pr correspond to P and pr' correspond to P'.

First let us apply Bayes Tautology in both situations:

$$pr(x_1|x_2) = pr(x_2|x_1)pr(x_1)/pr(x_2\}$$

$$pr'(x_1|x_2) = pr'(x_2|x_1)pr'(x_1)/pr'(x_2\}$$

The key assumption is that

$$pr(x_2|x_1) = pr'(x_2|x_1)$$

This means that even though the two sampling procedures might have differed, the above conditional distributions agree.

Although this situation might sound a bit unusual, it is in fact one of the primary methods of epidemiology. Here, x_2 is a cause of the disease x_1, as illustrated in Figure 1 on the left. The sampling procedure does not select opportunities at random. In fact, it first samples in the population of disease cases [$x_1=1$] and then samples separately in the population of non-cases [$x_1=0$]. When these two stratified samples are obtained, then one can compute the probability of the cause (x_2) in each of them, obtaining $pr'(x_2|x_1)$, which is indicated on the right in Figure 1. And here is where the assumption comes into play: this conditional distribution is the same as what one would have obtained if one had just sampled at random from the population of opportunities.

As an aside, the reason epidemiologists do this is to obtain parameter estimates with as little sampling variability as possible. Because most diseases are rare, whereas their causes are not, a random sample will turn up only a relatively small number of instances with disease and the cause, or disease without the cause. It is these small numbers that drive up the sampling variability of the odds ratio, the associational measure that epidemiologists prefer.

Since the causal parameters (on the left in Figure 1) reflect $pr(x_1|x_2)$, it is clear that they could be obtained in a study that performed stratified sampling with regard to x_2, under the assumptions discussed in Section 15. This is called a *prospective study*, because the conditional probability distribution is in the causal (and therefore, temporal) direction. The fundamental assumption behind this kind of study is that $pr(x_1|x_2)$ is the same as would have been obtained in a completely random sample, otherwise the probability model may be miss-specified for the causal parameters. Conversely, the sampling I described above, which is stratified by x_1, must have $pr'(x_2|x_1)$ the same as would have been obtained by a completely random sample, otherwise there is no connection between the right and left sides of Figure 1. Because the conditional distribution goes against the causal direction, this kind of study is called *retrospective*.

Prospective studies are usually regarded as not being particularly problematic, because the sample is actually obtained by something like

134

random sampling from a natural population of people. The fact that the cause is measured first, and then time passes, and finally the effect is measured, creates no sampling problems. Retrospective studies, on the other hand, require considerable care. If one does not obtain a random selection from among the cases [$x_1=1$], then there is no guarantee that the conditional distribution of the cause, given the effect, is the same as would be obtained in the corresponding prospective study. In describing retrospective studies, epidemiologists often place great emphasis on the fact that sampling from among the non-cases [$x_1=0$] must be properly random, and while this is certainly true, it tends to push the corresponding requirement for the cases into the background.

There is one kind of study, the "nested case-control" study in which this assumption is completely plausible. Here, one first samples from a natural population, and although the sample is followed up over time, no measurements are made. As cases of disease appear, they are inducted into the retrospective part of the study, and their x_2-values are measured. Usually each time a case appears, a non-case (at that time) is sampled at random, and likewise enters the retrospective study, and has their x_2-value measured. Because the sample was assembled at the start of the study, the identity of $pr(x_2|x_1)$ and $pr'(x_2|x_1)$ is all but assured. This design is especially attractive when measuring x_2 is expensive.

If the retrospective data is analyzed retrospectively, then the main analytic result that we need is

$$pr(x_1|x_2) = pr'(x_2|x_1)pr(x_1)/pr(x_2)$$

We obtain $pr'(x_2|x_1)$ by estimation (the retrospective part), obtain $pr(x_1)$ and $pr(x_2)$ from some other source (or by speculation; see below) and thus we convert the results of the right side of Figure 1 to the left side. The reversal equations of Section 20 are an example of this. It is often the case, however, that retrospective studies are analyzed prospectively. The justification is that if you are only interested in the odds ratio (which is all epidemiologists are interested in), then it doesn't make any difference whether you analyze prospectively or retrospectively. Thus, analyzing prospectively makes it possible to report retrospective studies in the same data format as would be used for prospective studies, and if simplification of the literature is your aim, then this looks attractive. The appropriate

135

analytic tool to go from right to left in Figure 1 is then the *double reversal* equation:

$$\text{pr}(x_1|x_2) = \text{pr}'(x_1|x_2) \frac{\text{pr}(x_1)\text{pr}'(x_2)}{\text{pr}'(x_1)\text{pr}(x_2)}$$

The left side is what we want (the left side of Figure 1), and the primed-elements on the right are what we will have. Again $\text{pr}'(x_1|x_2)$ is estimated by prospective analysis of the retrospective data, and we still need $\text{pr}(x_1)$ and $\text{pr}(x_2)$. Actually, we only require one of these. Usually $\text{pr}(x_1)$ is available, then summing both sides of the above equation over x_1 gives

$$\text{pr}(x_2) = \text{pr}'(x_2) \sum_{x_1} \text{pr}'(x_1|x_2) \frac{\text{pr}(x_1)}{\text{pr}'(x_1)}$$

For the computation of parameters, let us use $\xi_i = P[x_i=1]$ and $\xi'_i = P'[x_i=1]$. We then have

$$\beta^*_{1:02} = \beta^*_{2:0.1}\,\xi^*_1/\xi^*_2 = \beta'^*_{2:0.1}\,\xi^*_1/\xi^*_2 = \beta'^*_{1:0.2}\left(\xi^*_1\xi'^*_2\right)/\left(\xi^*_2\xi'^*_1\right)$$

The first equality is just ordinary reversal, and the second is due to the fundamental assumption $\text{pr}(x_2|x_1) = \text{pr}'(x_2|x_1)$. Thus, these two equations solve part of the problem in moving from the right to the left in Figure 1. The next equation now applies reversal again. This is one of the double reversal equations.

To obtain the second half of the double reversal equations, we follow the same path:

$$\beta_{1:2} = \beta_{2:1}\xi_1/\xi_2 = \beta'_{2:1}\xi_1/\xi_2 = \beta'_{1:2}(\xi_1\xi'_2)/(\xi_2\xi'_1)$$

and again the second equality would be used if the retrospective study were analyzed retrospectively, and the third equation would be used if it were analyzed prospectively.

In the usual case, ξ_1 will be known, and then the additional equation for ξ_2 is

$$\xi^*_2 = \xi'^*_2\left(\beta'^*_{1:0.2}\xi^*_1/\xi'^*_1 + \beta'_{1:0.2}\xi_1/\xi'_1\right)$$

For an example of this method, we turn to a retrospective study of women with cervical neoplasia on a PAP test, shown in prospective format in Table 1.

Oral Contraceptive Use	Probability of Neoplasia
No	$207/406 = 0.5099$
Yes	$117/220 = 0.5318$

Obstetrics and Gynecology 1972; 40(4):508-518 (Table 5, lines 7-8)

Table 1. Cervical neoplasia related to OC use.

We compute from the prospective analysis

$\beta'_{1:0.2} = 0.5099$

$\beta'_{1:2} = 0.5318 \setminus 0.5099 = 0.0447$

$\xi'_1 = (117+207)/(220+406) = 0.5176$

$\xi'_2 = 220/(220+406) = 0.3514$

For purposes of illustration, I will assume that $\xi_1 = 0.05$ in a prospective study in this population. We then compute

$\xi_2 = [\, 0.3514*(0.5099*0.05*/0.5176* + (0.5099)(0.05)/0.5176)]*$

$= 0.3420$

Finally, the causal parameters in the prospective study would have been

$\beta_{1:0.2} = [0.5099*(0.05*)(0.3520*)/(0.5176*)(0.3441*)]* = 0.0465$

$\beta_{1:2} = 0.0447(0.05)(0.3520)/(0.5176)(0.3441) = 0.0044$

The causal effect of OC use seen to be rather small; in a population where 50 women per thousand exhibit cervical neoplasia, the OC effect is 4.4 per thousand.

It should, perhaps be emphasized that the hypothetical prospective study (based on random sampling from the opportunities) would need to have a correctly specified model. If that model were miss-specified, then all of our adjustment of the retrospective results has merely been to obtain the wrong prospective causal effect estimate. In this case, that amounts to OC use being independent of residual causes of cervical neoplasia.

Although it is probably obvious, I also mention that the apparently causal results that would be computed from a prospective analysis of the retrospective study will virtually always be wrong. The double reversal procedure shows how to make them right.

Complex Indirect Cause

The purpose of this section is to show a few more examples of indirect cause, and to develop skills for computing parameters. The first example is shown in Figure 1. Here, x_4 causes both x_2 and x_3, and only causes x_1 through pathways that involve these two factors. x_2 and x_3 themselves cause x_1 directly. The problem is to compute the causal effect of x_4, but also to see how it is composed of the effects of various pathways.

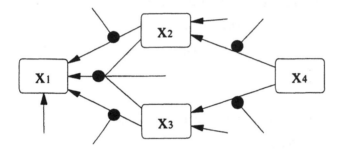

Figure 1. x_4 has only indirect effects on x_1 that act through x_2 and x_3.

One assumption is that the causal relationship $(x_2,x_3) \longrightarrow x_1$ [F] is correctly specified in the model

$$E[x_1|x_2,x_3,x_4] = \beta_{1:0.23} \vee \beta_{1:2.3}x_2 \vee \beta_{1:3.2}x_3 \vee \beta_{1:23}x_2x_3$$

Note that part of the assumption is that $x_1 \amalg x_4 \,|x_2,x_3$. Since there is no arrow between x_2 and x_3, another part of the assumption is that $x_2 \amalg x_3 \mid x_4$. This is the least satisfactory of the assumptions, since it restricts the cases in which we can apply the result we are about to derive. It is crucial, however, since it implies

$$E[x_2x_3|x_4] = E[x_2|x_4]E[x_3|x_4]$$

To see why this is important, let us do a little side computation. Assume

$$E[z_3|z_1,z_2] = \alpha_0 \vee \alpha_1 z_1 \vee \alpha_2 z_2 \vee \alpha_{12} z_1 z_2$$

and that $z_1 \amalg z_2$. Now letting $\zeta_i = E[z_i]$,

$$E[z_3] = E[\alpha_0 \vee \alpha_1 z_1 \vee \alpha_2 z_2 \vee \alpha_{12} z_1 z_2] =$$

$$E[\alpha_0 z_1^* z_2^* + (\alpha_0 \vee \alpha_1) z_1 z_2^* + (\alpha_0 \vee \alpha_2) z_1^* z_2 + (\alpha_0 \vee \alpha_1 \vee \alpha_2 \vee \alpha_{12}) z_1 z_2] =$$

$$= \alpha_0 \zeta_1^* \zeta_2^* + (\alpha_0 \vee \alpha_1) \zeta_1 \zeta_2^* + (\alpha_0 \vee \alpha_2) \zeta_1^* \zeta_2 + (\alpha_0 \vee \alpha_1 \vee \alpha_2 \vee \alpha_{12}) \zeta_1 \zeta_2 =$$

$$= (\alpha_0 \vee \alpha_1 \zeta_1) \zeta_2^* + (\alpha_0 \vee \alpha_2 \vee (\alpha_1 \vee \alpha_{12}) \zeta_1) \zeta_2 =$$

$$= \alpha_0 \vee \alpha_1 \zeta_1 \vee \{\alpha_0 \vee \alpha_2 \vee (\alpha_1 \vee \alpha_{12}) \zeta_1 \setminus (\alpha_0 \vee \alpha_1 \zeta_1)\} \zeta_2 =$$

$$= \alpha_0 \vee \alpha_1 \zeta_1 \vee \{\alpha_2 \vee \alpha_1 \zeta_1 \vee (\zeta_1 \setminus \alpha_1 \zeta_1) \alpha_{12} \setminus \alpha_1 \zeta_1\} \zeta_2 =$$

$$= \alpha_0 \vee \alpha_1 \zeta_1 \vee \alpha_2 \zeta_2 \vee (\zeta_1 \setminus \alpha_1 \zeta_1)(\zeta_2 \setminus \alpha_2 \zeta_2) \alpha_{12} =$$

$$= \alpha_0 \vee \alpha_1 \zeta_1 \vee \alpha_2 \zeta_2 \vee (\zeta_1 \downarrow \alpha_1)(\zeta_2 \downarrow \alpha_2) \alpha_{12}$$

where we have given in to the temptation to introduce the symbol $\downarrow$ meaning

$$u \downarrow v = u \setminus uv.$$

With this formula in hand, we can apply it to obtain

$$E[x_1|x_4] = E[E[x_1|x_2,x_3] \mid x_4] =$$

$$= \beta_{1:0.23} \vee \beta_{1:2.3} E[x_2|x_4] \vee \beta_{1:3.2} E[x_3|x_4]$$

$$\vee \beta_{1:23} (E[x_2|x_4] \downarrow \beta_{1:2.3})(E[x_3|x_4] \downarrow \beta_{1:3.2})$$

$$= \beta_{1:0.23} \vee \beta_{1:2.3}(\beta_{2:0.4} \vee \beta_{2:4} x_4) \vee \beta_{1:3.2}(\beta_{3:0.4} \vee \beta_{3:4} x_4)$$

$$\vee \beta_{1:23}((\beta_{2:0.4} \vee \beta_{2:4} x_4) \downarrow \beta_{1:2.3})((\beta_{3:0.4} \vee \beta_{3:4} x_4) \downarrow \beta_{1:3.2})$$

Substitution of $x_4 = 0$ gives

$$\beta_{1:0.4} = \beta_{1:0.23} \vee \beta_{1:2.3} \beta_{2:0.4} \vee \beta_{1:3.2} \beta_{3:0.4} \vee \beta_{1:23}(\beta_{2:0.4} \downarrow \beta_{1:2.3})(\beta_{3:0.4} \downarrow \beta_{1:3.2})$$

Substitution of $x_4 = 1$ and $\setminus$-subtracting $\beta_{1:0.4}$ gives

$$\beta_{1:4} = (\beta_{1:2.3} \downarrow \beta_{2:0.4}) \beta_{2:4} \vee (\beta_{1:3.2} \downarrow \beta_{3:0.4}) \beta_{3:4}$$

$$\vee \beta_{1:23}((\beta_{2:0.4} \vee \beta_{2:4}) \downarrow \beta_{1:2.3})((\beta_{3:0.4} \vee \beta_{3:4}) \downarrow \beta_{1:3.2})$$

$$\setminus \beta_{1:23}(\beta_{2:0.4} \downarrow \beta_{1:2.3})(\beta_{3:0.4} \downarrow \beta_{1:3.2})$$

Each of the terms that make up $\beta_{1:0.4}$ has a pathway interpretation. For example, $\beta_{1:2.3}\beta_{2:04}$ represents residual causes of x_2 that then directly cause x_1. The first two terms that compose $\beta_{1:4}$ are similarly interpretable. We have seen their form before, where a direct effect parameter (like $\beta_{1:2.3}$) is reduced due to residual pathways (to $\beta_{1:2.3}\downarrow\beta_{2:0.4}$) before multiplication by the remaining effect parameter ($\beta_{2:4}$). The final expression represents all effects through the joint x_2,x_3 pathways, net of the direct pathways, but obviously a more satisfying algebraic expression would be required to make this evident.

The next example is shown in Figure 2. Again the assumption is that the corresponding model is correctly specified, and that arrows not shown are not there. Notice that there is no arrow between x_3 and x_4, but that this has no impact on our computations because we will always condition on x_3 and x_4. Thus, this Figure could be taken to be agnostic about any relationships between these two factors, which is at slight variance with the "no arrows" convention.

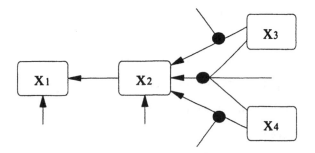

Figure 2. x_3 and x_4 cause x_1 only through their causation of x_2.

The conditional independence assumption of Figure 2 gives

$$E[x_1|x_2,x_3,x_4] = E[x_1|x_2]$$

and this justifies

$$E[x_1|x_3,x_4] = E[E[x_1|x_2] |x_3,x_4]$$

This in turn implies

$$\beta_{1:0.34} \vee \beta_{1:3.4} x_3 \vee \beta_{1:4.3} x_4 \vee \beta_{1:34} x_3 x_4 =$$

$$= \beta_{1:0.2} \vee \beta_{1:2}(\beta_{2:0.34} \vee \beta_{2:3.4} x_3 \vee \beta_{2:4.3} x_4 \vee \beta_{2:34} x_3 x_4)$$

Setting x_3 and x_4 to 0 gives

$$\beta_{1:0.34} = \beta_{1:0.2} \vee \beta_{1:2}\beta_{2:0.34}$$

Setting $x_3{=}1$ and $x_4{=}0$ gives

$$\beta_{1:0.34} \vee \beta_{1:3.4} = \beta_{1:0.2} \vee \beta_{1:2}(\beta_{2:0.34} \vee \beta_{2:3.4})$$

$$= \beta_{1:0.2} \vee \beta_{1:2}\beta_{2:0.34} \vee (\beta_{1:2} \!\downarrow\! \beta_{2:0.34})\beta_{2:3.4}$$

and so

$$\beta_{1:3.4} = (\beta_{1:2} \!\downarrow\! \beta_{2:0.34})\beta_{2:3.4}$$

By symmetric reasoning,

$$\beta_{1:4.3} = (\beta_{1:2} \!\downarrow\! \beta_{2:0.34})\beta_{2:4.3}$$

To ease the notation a little, let us use $\alpha = \beta_{1:2} \!\downarrow\! \beta_{2:0.34}$ in what follows, because it occurs so often. Now setting both x_3 and x_4 to 1 gives

$$\beta_{1:0.43} \vee \beta_{1:3.4} \vee \beta_{1:4.3} \vee \beta_{1:34} = \beta_{1:0.2} \vee \beta_{1:2}(\beta_{2:0.34} \vee \beta_{2:3.4} \vee \beta_{2:4.3} \vee \beta_{2:34}) =$$

$$= \beta_{1:0.34} \vee \alpha(\beta_{2:3.4} \vee \beta_{2:4.3} \vee \beta_{2:34}) =$$

$$= \beta_{1:0.34} \vee \alpha(\beta_{2:3.4} \vee \beta_{2:4.3}) \vee (\alpha \!\downarrow\! (\beta_{2:3.4} \vee \beta_{2:4.3})\beta_{2:34})$$

To take the next step it is convenient to derive

$$u(v \vee w) = uv \vee uw \vee (v \!\downarrow\! u)(w \!\downarrow\! u)(\backslash u)$$

so that we can proceed

$$\ldots = \beta_{1:0.34} \vee \alpha\beta_{2:3.4} \vee \alpha\beta_{2:4.3} \vee (\beta_{2:3.4} \!\downarrow\! \alpha)(\beta_{2:4.3} \!\downarrow\! \alpha)(\backslash\alpha))$$

$$\vee (\alpha \!\downarrow\! (\beta_{2:3.4} \vee \beta_{2:4.3})\beta_{2:34})$$

Therefore,

$$\beta_{1:34} = (\beta_{2:3.4} \!\downarrow\! \alpha)(\beta_{2:4.3} \!\downarrow\! \alpha)(\backslash\alpha)) \vee (\alpha \!\downarrow\! (\beta_{2:3.4} \vee \beta_{2:4.3})\beta_{2:34})$$

It is, of course, dismaying that even fairly simple "complex" models lead to such elaborate computations. On the one hand, we may rely on the fact that nature does not necessarily organize herself so that our understanding of her will be simple, and on the other hand, there may well be ways to simplify the unitary algebra that I have not thought of.

Dual Causation: Probabilities

Dual causation refers to the situation in which both x $\longrightarrow$ y [F] and x* $\longrightarrow$ y* [F]. That is, x is a cause of y, and the absence of x is a cause of the absence of y. In this section I assume that the probability models implied by these causal relations are correctly specified. Thus, I can write

$$P[y=1|x] = \beta_0 \vee \beta_1 x$$

$$P[y^*=1|x^*] = \alpha_0 \vee \alpha_1 x^*$$

and the parameters have their causal interpretations.

Dual causation does not appear as a concept in most of the literature on causation. One can understand this in the philosophical literature, since few causal theorists rely on a base of causal logic, but it is somewhat surprising that the idea has not made more progress among empirical scientists. The causal diagrams and models in the social sciences are oblivious to dual causation because of the probability models that they have chosen to use. In epidemiology, however, where the dominant trend has been to think in terms of factors (even when there is a better, underlying continuous measurement), the failure to appreciate dual causation is particularly hard to understand.

Another reason why it is problematic historically is that Mindel Sheps had already in her 1958 paper[1] presented a classic example of dual causation. She used the national field trial of the poliomyelitis vaccine carried out in the 1950's. Here x = lack of vaccination and y = polio. The causal relation x $\longrightarrow$ y [F] says that lack of vaccination is a cause of polio, and the causal relation x* $\longrightarrow$ y* [F] says that vaccination prevents polio. Although it is natural to focus on the latter relation (as Sheps herself did), both viewpoints are valid and worthwhile. Again assuming that the results of the vaccine trial led to correctly specified models, Sheps computed

$$P[y=1|x] = 0.00016 \vee (0.00057 \setminus 0.00016)x$$

$$= 0.00016 \vee 0.00040x$$

$$P[y^*=1|x^*] = 0.00057 \lor (0.99984 \setminus 0.99943)x^*$$
$$= 0.00057 \lor 0.71930x^*$$

The latter equation shows a more impressive effect of vaccination as a preventive, which is perhaps why the Centers for Disease Control and Prevention in the United States prefers it as a measure of immunization efficacy. But the first equation is equally valid, and of public health significance.

Returning to the dual causation model equations, we can compute that

$$P[y=1|x=0] = \beta_0 = P[y^*=0|x^*=1] = \alpha_0^*\alpha_1^*$$
$$P[y^*=1|x^*=0] = \alpha_0 = P[y=0|x=1] = \beta_0^*\beta_1^*$$

This suggests that we ought to be able to express α_0 and β_0 in terms of α_1 and β_1. Write

$$\beta_0 = \alpha_0^*\alpha_1^* = (\beta_0 \lor \beta_1)\alpha_1^* = (\beta_1 + \beta_1^*\beta_0)\alpha_1^*$$

and then solving for β_0

$$\beta_0 = \beta_1\alpha_1^*/(\alpha_1^*\beta_1^*)^* = (\alpha_1/(\alpha_1 \lor \beta_1))^*$$

A symmetric argument works for α_0 and so the assumption of the IFR for the dual causation equations leads to

$$P[y=1|x] = (\alpha_1/(\alpha_1 \lor \beta_1))^* \lor \beta_1 x$$
$$P[y^*=1|x^*] = (\beta_1/(\beta_1 \lor \alpha_1))^* \lor \alpha_1 x^*$$

realizing the suspicion that α_1 and β_1 are the only free parameters.

The probabilistic dual causation equations will not carry us very far, and a more complex consideration of this phenomenon will be given in the next Section. There is, however, a very interesting consequence that is of considerable importance for understanding the causal implications of most modern epidemiologic studies. In these studies, it is established that the measure of association between a potential cause of disease and the disease itself is the odds ratio, defined by

$$OR = \frac{P[y = 1|x = 1]P[y = 0|x = 0]}{P[y = 1|x = 0]P[y = 0|x = 1]}$$

where y is the disease and x is the potential cause. By direct substitution

$$OR = \frac{(\beta_0 \vee \beta_1)\beta_0^*}{\beta_0(\beta_0 \vee \beta_1)^*} = \frac{\beta_0 \vee \beta_1}{\beta_0\beta_1^*} = \frac{\alpha_0^*}{\alpha_0^*\alpha_1^*\beta_1^*} = \frac{1}{(\alpha_1 \vee \beta_1)^*}$$

Or expressed slightly differently,

$$(OR-1)/OR = \alpha_1 \vee \beta_1$$

This shows that the odds ratio is a combination of two different causal effects, the effect of x in causing y (β_1) and the effect of x* in causing y* (α_1). In other words, the harmful effects of x are confounded with the preventive effects of x* in the odds ratio.

The causal implications of this cannot be over-emphasized. Epidemiologists and biostatisticians who have promoted the use of the odds ratio have done so without having established the relationship of this measure to an underlying causal theory. The result has been an associational measure that, whatever its virtues, has failed to distinguish between two fundamentally different causal processes. It is a mark of the success of the minimal sufficient cause approach to have separated these two aspects of causation.

Reference

1. Sheps, MC. Shall we count the living or the dead? *New England Journal of Medicine* 1958;259:1210-1214

Dual Causation: Structures

In the preceding section I was only concerned with the probability models implied by dual causation. Here I want to look at the underlying structural equations in some detail. To continue the notation of the preceding section, I have two equations

$$C[y|F] = b_0 \vee b_1 x \qquad \text{causal}[F]$$

$$C[y^*|F] = a_0 \vee a_1 x^* \qquad \text{causal}[F]$$

As I have done before, for convenience of notation I assume (with no real loss of generality) that y and y^* are in $\vee\Pi F$.

All possible values of the relevant factors are shown in Table 1. The two $y|x$ columns give the value of y, depending on which value x takes. In general, one might imagine that all possible values of b_0, a_0, b_1, a_1, and x could be assumed. Under some combinations, however, y must be both zero and one, given the dual causation equations. These disallowed situations are denoted by ✻ in the table.

The idea that some logical possibilities are not actually possible is an inevitable consequence of the existence of multiple causal relationships, all of which must be satisfied simultaneously. This phenomenon has been implicit in causal diagrams we have seen before, but here we have the first instance in which the causal relationships restrict the possible combinations of the values of the causal field in quite this way. Thus, for instance, the equation $a_0 b_0 = 0$ is forced by the dual causal equations, and this explains why the last four rows in Table 1 are disallowed.

A further interesting pattern emerges if we suppose that b_0, a_0, b_1, and a_1 are *traits*. This means that no other causal laws can change their values. Consequently, these factors are fixed for each opportunity. We might then suppose that x is a *state*, which means that for each opportunity ω, it could happen that either $x(\omega) = 0$, or $x(\omega) = 1$, and this might change due to other causal laws. For humans, gender is regarded as a trait, since (with rare exceptions) it does not change throughout life, but body weight is a state, because it can (and does) vary over the lifespan.

b_0	b_1	a_0	a_1	$y\vert x=0$	$y\vert x=1$	T
1	0	0	0	1	1	✓
1	0	0	1	*	1	
1	1	0	0	1	1	✓
1	1	0	1	*	1	
0	0	1	0	0	0	✓
0	0	1	1	0	0	✓
0	1	1	0	0	*	
0	1	1	1	0	*	
0	0	0	0	*	*	
0	0	0	1	0	*	
0	1	0	0	*	1	
0	1	0	1	0	1	✓
1	0	1	0	*	*	
1	0	1	1	*	*	
1	1	1	0	*	*	
1	1	1	1	*	*	

Table 1. All possible combinations of factors. *
indicates a situation not allowed by dual causation.
The T column shows which rows are allowed if the
a's and b's are traits but x is a state.

Some versions of causation require that changes in the cause somehow
produce changes in the effect. For example, a key feature of Rubin's
approach to causation (see Section 28) is that as scientific investigators we
can make the cause either 0 or 1, for any individual. This is the same as
saying that the cause must be a state, and cannot be a trait.

By writing the tautology

$$0 = y^*y = a_0b_0 \vee a_0b_1x \vee b_0a_1x^*$$

we can see that when x is a state, we must have $a_0b_1=0$ and $b_0a_1=0$. When
we eliminate the rows in Table 1 that violate these conditions, we are left
with those having a ✓ under the T column. These are the only possible
rows in a world where the a's and b's are traits and x is a state. This
illustrates one role of causation, that causal rules narrow the range of
possibilities in any world that is free of causal contradictions.

The trait/state assumption has a very interesting consequence. By
inspection of Table 1, we can see that the only row checked under T
where x makes any difference to the effect is row 12. This row is

148

equivalent to [$a_1 b_1 = 1$], again among the checked rows. As a consequence, if we define $c = a_1 b_1$ then the causal equations become

$$y = b_0 \lor cx \qquad \text{causal}[F]$$

$$y^* = a_0 \lor cx^* \qquad \text{causal}[F]$$

In other words, there is a distinct set of opportunities that are susceptible to the causal effect of x; the remainder are immune. A bit of thought shows that $a_0 + b_0 + c = 1$, a partition of Ω.

It is worth noting that we can have the IFR in both causal equations ($x \longrightarrow y$ [F] and $x^* \longrightarrow y^*$ [F]). The rows deleted from Table 1 do not prevent independence of cause and residual, and even if we make the trait/state assumptions that disallow further columns, the IFR is still possible. Thus, the discussion of the probability models in the preceding Section was not vacuous.

One will want to invoke the dual causation assumption only after some consideration. For example, it appears to make sense to say that cigarette smoking causes certain diseases, in part because we can trace some mechanistic causal pathways, at least for some diseases. It seems to make less sense, however, to say that the absence of smoking causes the absence of these diseases. Not smoking is hard to view as a specific factor with well-defined characteristics, since some non-cigarette-smokers are vegetarian exercise enthusiasts while others are cigar-smoking alcohol abusers, which strains the notion that there is some underlying factor here. This explains, by the way, why I did not require that F (or ΠF, or $\lor \Pi F$) be closed under complementation. It also provides an additional argument against using the odds ratio as a measure of causal force.

Note further that we have the mathematical equation

$$y^* = b_0^* b_1^* \lor b_0^* x^*$$

but by inspection of Table 1, this is not a causal equation, even if we admitted the complementary factors into F. This provides another example of a case in which there is a distinction between mathematical and causal equations.

In graphical representations, note that we require two arrows to denote the dual causal relationship, as in Figure 1.

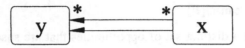

Figure 1. Two arrows are required to show dual causation.

To illustrate a more complex case, consider Figure 2. Here the implied causal structural equations are

$$y = b_{0.12} \vee b_{1.2}x_1 \vee b_{2.1}x_2 \vee b_{12}x_1x_2$$

$$y^* = a_{0.12} \vee a_{1.2}x_1{}^* \vee a_{12}x_1{}^*x_2$$

and it should be obvious why we do not even attempt to represent the a's and b's in the diagram.

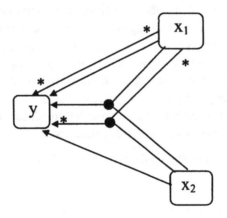

Figure 2. x_1 is a dual cause of y, along pathways unique to it as well as pathways shared with x_2.

Paradoxical Causation

Paradoxical causation occurs when both a factor and its complement cause the same effect. On initial reflection, one might think that this must occur rarely, if at all. There are, however, enough examples that we believe we understand to suggest that it warrants treatment by any viable causal theory.

A general example is immunization using a killed- or attenuated-virus vaccine against an infectious disease y. We would usually say that x = "absence of vaccination" is a cause of y, since individuals not naturally immune, who come into contact with the virus, become diseased if they were not vaccinated. It is possible, however, that some of those who are vaccinated ($x^*=1$) are exposed to vaccine that is not sufficiently attenuated, relative to their immune systems, so that they acquire the disease directly from the immunization. (There was some evidence in the national field trial of the Salk polio vaccine in the US in the 1950's that vaccination with a placebo could very slightly raise the disease rate, so that the injection itself might cause some cases.)

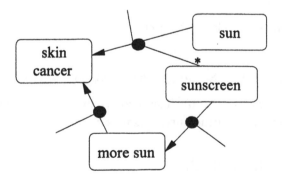

Figure 1. Although sunscreen usually blocks the effect of sunlight, it can also cause increased sun exposure.

A less obvious example is shown in Figure 1. It is widely believed that sun exposure is a cause of skin cancer. A sunscreen is a cream to be applied to sun-exposed skin surfaces, which is supposed to capture some of the energy from sunlight before it can penetrate the epidermis, and cause mutations in the cells that reside there. Thus, sunscreen prevents skin cancer by preventing cancer-causing mutations. It is possible, however, that some people who use sunscreen chose to expose themselves to even more sun, in the false hope that the sunscreen has no limit in its ability to absorb light energy. Since the additional sun exposure swamps the sunscreen's protective effect, the result is carcinogenic mutations. This means that sunscreen can also be a cause of skin cancer.

There are some other not-so-obvious examples. A medication that clearly suppressed cardiac arrythmias in most people evidently induced them in others, leading to its being withdrawn from use.[1] Caffeine is a stimulant for most people, but among certain hyper-active children the absence of caffeine could be seen as a cause of the over-stimulation. On reflection, paradoxical causation is more common than we might think.

The paradoxical causal equation is (again assuming for notational convenience that $y = C[y|F]$)

$$y = b_{0.12} \vee b_{1.2}x \vee b_{2.1}x^* \qquad \text{causal}[F]$$

where I have identified x_1 with x and x_2 with x^*, and both are assumed members of F. Of course, $b_{12} = 0$ on account of $x^*x = 0$. The probability model that follows from this is simpler than it is in the general case. First, note that we can write

$$P[\text{anything}|x, x^*] = P[\text{anything}|x]$$

Then

$$P[b_{0.12} = 1|x] = \beta_{0.12} \vee \delta_{0.1}x \vee \delta_{0.2}x^* = \beta_{0.12} \vee \delta_{0.2} \vee (\delta_{0.1} \backslash \delta_{0.2})x$$

(again $\delta_{0.12} = 0$ because $x^*x = 0$). The second equation shows that we can set $\delta_{0.2} = 0$ without loss of generality. Again due to $x^*x = 0$ we automatically have

$$P[b_{1.2} = 1|x = 1, b_{0.12} = 0] = \beta_{1.2}$$

$$P[b_{2.1} = 1|x^* = 1, b_{0.12} = 0] = \beta_{2.1}$$

The δ_{12} parameter is undefined, and so finally

$$P[y = 1|x] = \beta_{0.12} \vee (\beta_{1.2} \vee \delta_{0.1})x \vee \beta_{2.1}x^* =$$

$$= \beta_{0.12} \vee \beta_{2.1} \vee ((\beta_{1.2} \backslash \beta_{2.1}) \vee \delta_{0.1}) x$$

Now IFR in this case means $x \amalg b_{0.12}$, or equivalently $\delta_{0.1} = 0$, but even this condition will not permit estimation of the causal effect of x, which is $\beta_{1.2}$, nor that of x^*, which is $\beta_{2.1}$. The naïve computation of the causal effect of x will be $\beta_{1.2} \backslash \beta_{2.1}$, which must understate the true effect, and may possibly even reverse its sign.

What is happening here is that the causal parameters are well defined, but they are not determined by the probability distributions. In a sense we can see this by just counting. We only have two pieces of information in $P[y=1|x]$, but there are three parameters, $\beta_{0.12}$, $\beta_{1.2}$, and $\beta_{2.1}$. No amount of observation (of this type) will solve the problem.

One potential solution would be to find factors x_3 and x_4 such that x acted only through x_3 and x^* acted only through x_4. This would give us the situation of Figure 2. If we can compute the causal parameters in $(x_3, x_4) \longrightarrow y$ [F], $x \longrightarrow x_3$ [F], and $x^* \longrightarrow x_4$ [F], then we can use our unitary algebra skills to obtain $\beta_{0.12}$, $\beta_{1.2}$ and $\beta_{2.1}$.

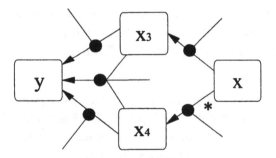

Figure 2. The paradoxical causation problem can be solved by finding the separate pathways through which x and x^* act.

There is another example that is not exactly paradoxical, but has some of the same flavor. Suppose that there is a genetic locus at which an active allele may or may not be present. Let x_1 denote the event that an individual receives the active allele from the father, and x_2 similarly from the mother. Now suppose that either two active alleles or two inactive

153

alleles both cause disease. This is called a balanced polymorphism, and it actually occurs. The causal equation would be

$$y = b_{12}x_1x_2 \vee b_{34}x_1{}^*x_2{}^*$$

where I am playing a little loose with the notation, but thinking of $x_1{}^*$ as x_3 and $x_2{}^*$ as x_4. In this genetics example it is reasonable to assume that x_1 and x_2 are independent. We let $E[x_1] = \xi_1$ and $E[x_2] = \xi_2$, although again in the genetics example it would be reasonable to take $\xi_1 = \xi_2$. Finally, I assume that the corresponding probability model is correctly specified for β_{12} and β_{34}.

Now the interesting result that follows from this is

$$P[y=1|x_1] = \beta_{34}\xi_2{}^* \vee (\beta_{12}\xi_2 \setminus \beta_{34}\xi_2{}^*)x_1$$

It is easy to check that if $\xi_2 = \beta_{34}/(\beta_{12}+\beta_{34})$ then the above expression does not depend on x_1. This shows a realistic situation in which x_1 is a cause of y, but y is independent of x_1, again illustrating the fact that causation does not imply association. For general values of ξ_2, it is clear that y could appear more positively related to x_1 as x_2 becomes more prevalent, but that y could actually be negatively related to x_1 if x_2 were sufficiently rare.

On reflection, there is an even more troubling example along these lines (although it does not happen to be a realistic genetic example). Suppose that $\beta_{12} = \beta_{34} = 1$ and $\xi_1 = \xi_2 = \frac{1}{2}$. Then

$$y = x_1x_2 \vee x_1{}^*x_2{}^*$$

so that y is a deterministic function of x_1 and x_2, yet $y \amalg x_1$ and $y \amalg x_2$. This is a physically realizable model (see Figure 5 in Section 9). If there is any situation that should make one think twice before trying to define causation in terms of association, surely this is it.

Reference

1. Moore TJ. Deadly Medicine. New York NY: Simon & Schuster, 1995.

Interventions

Many, if not most scientific theories of causation are given in terms of changes. The idea can be expressed in an astonishingly different number of ways, but it all comes down to saying that a change in x in some sense produces a change in y. In medical research it is virtually an article of faith that one can only begin to demonstrate causality if one "intervenes" by producing changes. The definition of an *intervention* is that the researchers cause a particular change, rather than that change having been produced by some other causal law.

Taking an intervention as the necessary touchstone of a causal demonstration is an example of a circular argument. If a change in x causes a change in y only when the change in x is caused by the investigators, then what is the definition of a change *caused by the investigators*? I will not go down this path, but rather simply consider what are some of the consequences of trying to think about cause in terms of change.

Rubin's Theory. One causal theory based on change is due to Rubin[1,2,3]. He posits that each opportunity in Ω is associated with two factors, $\eta(0,\omega)$ and $\eta(1,\omega)$. These factors are occult, and they exist before the experiment is performed. The resulting observed value of y will be $y(\omega) = \eta(x(\omega),\omega)$. We may call the η's the *hypothetical response profile* or *HRP*. It is a listing of the responses that will be made, depending on which value is taken by the cause x. Reality is simply determined by plugging the causal effect into the HRP, so that this is a functional definition of causation, with each opportunity having its own causal function.

There are some philosophical problems with Rubin's approach that usually go under the title "counterfactual arguments." The reason for the nomenclature is that after the experiment we get to see $\eta(x(\omega),\omega)$, but not $\eta(x^*(\omega),\omega)$. We can then think of $\eta(x^*(\omega),\omega)$ as the effect that *would have* happened *if* x *had been* the opposite of what it was. Since this description posits things that did not happen, philosophers call it "counterfactual". The great problem with counterfactuals is that it is not sufficient to say just "x was the opposite of what it was". We have to say what else might differ in this counterfactual world, and until we do, there is some intolerable ambiguity. I will go down this path, but only insofar as it affects a world created by a very small number of factors, shown in Table 1.

$b_{0.1}$	b_1^i	b_1^d	a_1	$\eta(0)$	$\eta(1)$
0	0	0	0	0	0
0	0	0	1	*	*
0	0	1	0	0	1
0	0	1	1	*	*
0	1	0	0	0	?
0	1	0	1	*	*
0	1	1	0	0	?
0	1	1	1	*	*
1	0	0	0	1	1
1	0	0	1	1	?
1	0	1	0	1	1
1	0	1	1	1	1
1	1	0	0	1	1
1	1	0	1	1	1
1	1	1	0	1	1
1	1	1	1	1	1

Table 1. All possible values of factors with their corresponding HRPs. * means disallowed, ? means that the value cannot be determined without further assumptions.

One of these factors is the residual cause, $b_{0.1}$. Two of the others are the indirect and direct co-causes, as defined in Section 19. The last is the co-cause in the causal relation $x_1 \longrightarrow b_1$ [F]. I call this a_1, and it is defined by

$$a_1 = \vee \{f \in \Pi F_1 : fx_1 \overset{s}{\longrightarrow} b_1, f \overset{s}{\longmapsto} b_1\}$$

All logical combinations of these factors are shown in Table 1, along with the HRP. I am going to make the innocuous assumption that

156

$C[b_1|F]=b_1$. Recall this means that all of the causes of b_1 are in F, which in principle I should be able to attain by making F big enough. It then follows that four of the logically possible rows cannot happen, because $a_1 \leq b_{0.1}$. This is shown as follows. Let f satisfy the definition of a_1. Then $fx_1 \xrightarrow{\text{NT}} b_1 \Rightarrow fx_1 \xrightarrow{\text{NT}} b_1 x_1 \xrightarrow{\text{T}} y \Rightarrow fx_1 \xrightarrow{\text{T}} y$. Now if $f \xrightarrow{\text{T}} y$ then f would satisfy the definition of b_1, and so $f \xrightarrow{\text{NT}} b_1 = C[b_1|F] \xrightarrow{\text{T}} b_1$, a contradiction. Thus $f \xrightarrow{\text{T}} y$, finishing the demonstration.

Two of the rows in the second block of Table 1 have ? for $\eta(1)$. This is because when $x_1=1$ we have

$$b_1^i x_1 = 1, \ b_{0.1} = 0$$

contradicting the causal equation for $b_{0.1}$. Something has to change, in order for this causal equation to be preserved. One possibility is that x_1 could be prohibited from being 1. This would be the only possibility if the b's and a_1 were traits (see Section 26). Rubin assumes, however, as a fundamental part of his theory, that x_1 can assume either of the values 0 or 1 for each opportunity; in other words, no values of x_1 can be prohibited. I will continue here with this assumption, even though it is not an assumption of MSC. Now in order to preserve all causal equations, either $b_{0.1}$ must change to 1 or b_1^i must change to 0 in the above circumstances. It follows immediately that there must be a factor which indicates which of these alternatives will happen. Although it is possible for both $b_{0.1}$ and b_1^i to change simultaneously, since only one change is necessary to preserve the causal equations, we might presume that they never both change.

This shows that if the situations of rows 5 and 7 in Table 1 occur, then there exists a factor f_1 such that in cases where $x_1=1$ in those rows, we must have

change $b_{0.1}$ to $b_{0.1} \vee f_1$

change b_1^i to $b_1^i f_1$

and we can take $f_1=0$ for all other rows and cases where $x_1=0$. This leads to two equally unhappy possibilities. First, if $f_1 \notin \vee \Pi F_1$ then neither of the changed $b_{0.1}$ or b_1^i need to be members of $\vee \Pi F_1$ either, which violates their definitions. On the other hand, if $f_1 \in \vee \Pi F_1$, then since $f_1 \xrightarrow{\text{NT}} x_1$ we have a difficulty with the assumption that the investigators are free to set the value of x_1. Consequently, if we are going to continue with Rubin's basic assumptions, lines 5 and 7 of Table 1 cannot occur.

The remaining problem row is in the third block of Table 1, and here the ? denotes a case in which $b_1 = b_1 \vee a_1 x_1$ is violated. This again requires a new factor, say f_2, indicating that one (or both) of the indirect or direct co-cause changes to 1 in this case, thereby changing b_1 to 1. Again we can take f_2 to be 0 for all other rows and all cases where $x_1=0$. But f_2 now creates exactly the same problems that f_1 did in the preceding paragraph, so again if we are going to keep Rubin company, we must declare the row 10 in Table 1 as excluded.

To summarize the situation so far, in order for MSC and Rubin's definitions to co-exist, Table 1 must be reduced to the possibilities shown in Table 2.

$b_{0.1}$	b_1^i	b_1^d	a_1	$\eta(0)$	$\eta(1)$
0	0	0	0	0	0
0	0	1	0	0	1
1	0	0	0	1	1
1	0	1	0	1	1
1	0	1	1	1	1
1	1	0	0	1	1
1	1	0	1	1	1
1	1	1	0	1	1
1	1	1	1	1	1

Table 2. All possible values of factors with their corresponding HRPs if one assumes both MSC and Rubin's conditions.

There is only one case left in Table 2 in which Rubin would say that x_1 can cause a change, the second row. Here the only co-cause of x_1 is its direct co-cause. We conclude that no cause that is part of an indirect causal pathway (in the MSC sense) will satisfy Rubin's definition of being a cause. This is true because Rubin's assumptions eliminate three of the twelve possible rows of Table 1; that is, his assumptions impose occult conditions on reality, from the MSC viewpoint.

As I took some care to point out in Section 1, I am not interested in attacking Rubin's approach, particularly because it can be used to derive some extremely useful results. I must note, however, that his fundamental

158

assumptions appear to struggle with the MSC approach to a very considerable extent. Rubin's proponents[3] have said that it must be possible for x to change *at every opportunity* ω for there to be any question of causation. In addition to cases where x is a trait, this also rules out even the simplest MSC causal relationships when the factors shown in Table 1 are traits. Moreover, even when they are states, Rubin's approach implicitly assumes the impossibility of situations that are allowed by MSC.

Even if we were to work our way around these difficulties, another real problem here is that it will not always be possible to define the intervention in such a way that it changes x *and nothing else*. As we have seen, what else must be changed (or excluded) is not determined without additional causal conditions. In this way, the MSC approach explains precisely the sense in which the counterfactuality of Rubin's definition is problematic. In the end, it appears that without some additional insights or refinements, the MSC approach and Rubin's HRP will be extremely difficult to harmonize.

These problems have been addressed by Rubin, in the form of his "stable unit treatment value assumption" (SUTVA). One consequence of this assumption is that x cannot affect (Rubin's word) the HRP. This would seem to require $b_1^i = 0$ and $a_1 = 0$ in the above development, again consisting of additional constraints not imposed by MSC.

Counterfactuality. It may be useful to see a less technical example that gives some insight into the problem with counterfactuals. In Figure 1 we see a schematic in which person A points a gun at B, pulls the trigger, and the bullet strikes B both killing him and causing him to fall backwards. An instant after A fires, person C also fires at B, but because he is a lousy shot, C aims behind B's original position. C's bullet also hits B, but because B is already dead, C's bullet does not kill him. This narrative is based on our commonsense understanding of causation, and describes what actually happened. Presumably everyone would say that A caused B's death.

How could we establish this by a counterfactual argument? According to this method of reasoning we would have to say that if A had not fired, then *in the circumstances* B would not have died. The phrase "in the circumstances" is philosophy code for saying that the only thing

159

that changed is A's not firing, and this had no other (relevant) causal effects. Well then, in particular B must have fallen backward anyway, and so C's bullet would have killed him. Thus, if A had not fired *in the circumstances* then B would have died. In the counterfactual sense, A did not kill B.

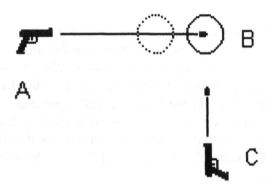

Figure 1. A fires at B, both killing him and moving him into C's line of fire. Commonsense says A killed B, but the counterfactual argument says not.

One is tempted to say that the problem is a compound counterfactual, in the sense that the *in the circumstances* phrase is counterfactual, or else there was some hidden factor that caused B to fall backwards, reminiscent of the shifting causal field problem. It should be relatively easy to see that in more complex situations counterfactual arguments are likely to become increasing tortuous.

Practical Interventions. The rationales for investigator-interventions that are given in practice are considerably less theoretical than Rubin's. They tend to sound as though the intervention is something outside of the causal system, which acts upon it, rather than being part of the causal system itself. To see what this means, consider Figure 2, which depicts a typical disease prevention study. Left on its own, this causal system says that "behavior" is a cause of the absence of "disease". The study injects two new factors into the picture, "treatment" and "on study". The intent of the investigators is that those people randomized to the "treatment" will be caused to activate "behavior" which then will prevent "disease".

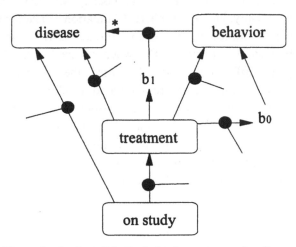

Figure 2. In the wild, the behavior prevents the disease. The intervention study introduces new factors, whose causal role must be understood.

Of course "treatment" could cause "behavior" only indirectly, by causing its residual cause, but that would not lessen its usefulness. "Treatment" could, however, cause the co-cause of "behavior", and this would be more serious. As we have seen, the apparent force of a cause depends on how plentiful is its co-cause. Increasing the frequency of the co-cause does, indeed, make the cause more powerful. But this is not an effect achieved by causing the "behavior" itself, opening the possibility that the nature of the beneficial effect of treatment might be misunderstood. If the study is successful, and therefore a public program is undertaken to increase "behavior", the observed effect on "disease*" may be much less than expected if the public health version of the intervention does not also cause the co-cause of "behavior". There is further the possibility that "treatment" causes "disease*" along pathways that do not involve "behavior". Finally, one must consider that "treatment" itself is caused by selection to be in the study (the "on study" variable), and since this factor will not be present in the public health

161

intervention, its effects will not be felt, although they may have been unintentionally included in the analysis of the prevention study.

The "no intervention - no cause" approach, whether stated philosophically or practically, has some inherent limitations. The concept of an HRP is extremely attractive, and almost sounds as if no special assumptions need be made to invoke it. But when put next to the MSC structure, unanticipated difficulties arise. Likewise, the commonsense idea of investigator intervention in a controlled, randomized trial, has very much caught the attention and approval of the medical community, but once again there are causal aspects that should be considered even in studies that have been well-conducted by conventional standards. It is a virtue of the MSC approach that it brings these issues into the open, and provides a language and framework for discussing them.

References

1. Rubin DB. Estimating causal effects of treatments in randomized and nonrandomized studies. *Journal of Educational Psychology* 1974;66:688-701

2. Rubin DB. Bayesian inference for causal effects: the role of randomization. *Annals of Statistics* 1978;6:34-58

3. Holland PW. Statistics and causal inference. *Journal of the American Statistical Association* 1986;81:945-960

Causal Covariance

Analogy with Regression. The structural causal equation $y = b_0 \lor b_1 x$ [F] and its probability counterpart $E[y|x] = \beta_0 \lor \beta_1 x$ (assuming IFR) are obviously intended to mimic the phenomenally useful linear regression model $y = \alpha_0 + \alpha_1 x + e$ and its probability form $E[y|x] = \alpha_0 + \alpha_1 x$. Indeed, the only difference between the two is the use of unitary vs. usual addition. I hope by now the reader will appreciate some of the virtues of using unitary algebra for binary causal equations.

But just in case this has not yet happened, let us consider for a moment what the consequences would be, if we used linear regression for our binary factors. The fundamental assumption about the "e" term in the regression equation is that it is uncorrelated with x. Without this condition, there is no possibility of going any further. This presents no problem. It is curious, however, that e cannot be *independent* of x except in the special case when $\alpha_1 = 0$. This is because the only possible values that can be assumed by e are $-\alpha_0$ and $1-\alpha_0$ when x=0, or $-\alpha_0 - \alpha_1$ and $1-\alpha_0-\alpha_1$ when x=1, but in order for it to be independent of x, the range of possible values of e must not depend on x.

The second way in which the linear regression model fights with binary factors is that the distribution of e is supposed to be free of the α-parameters. As we have just seen, to the contrary the very values that e can assume depend on the α-parameters.

The conclusion is that while the linear regression model has substantial virtues for variables that can be measured on a continuous scale, it is strained when applied to factors. One of the purposes of this book has been to try to develop models for measuring causation as a consequence of the structural form of the underlying causal relationships, rather than to select a mathematical model due to its convenient statistical properties, and then somehow hope that nature will go along with it.

Definition & Properties. Nevertheless, just as the causal probability model mimics the regression model, we might look for some other analogies between the two approaches. In linear modeling, an important role is played by the covariance between two stochastic variables, defined by

$$cov(x,y) = E[xy] - E[x]E[y]$$

I will assume that the reader is familiar with this measure. The causal analog of this that I would like to introduce is the *causal covariance*,

$$ccov(x,y) = E[x] \vee E[y] \setminus E[x \vee y].$$

The remainder of this section is designed to show some features of this measure, and to relate these to the corresponding properties of cov.

First, note that from

$$E[x] \vee E[y] = E[x] + E[y] - E[x]E[y]$$

$$E[x \vee y] = E[x] + E[y] - E[xy]$$

we have

$$ccov(x,y) = cov(x,y)/E[x \vee y]^*$$

From this we immediately conclude that $x \amalg y \Leftrightarrow ccov(x,y)=0$.

It might not be an exaggeration to say that the most useful property of the usual covariance is

$$cov(x,y) = cov(E[x|z],E[y|z]) + E[cov(x,y|z)]$$

Indeed, this formula is the basis for all of the computations involving "path coefficients" in the linear causal models that are used in the social sciences. The corresponding equation for the causal covariance is a little more complex:

$$ccov(x,y) = ccov(E[x|z],E[y|z]) \vee E[ccov(x,y|z)\{E[x \vee y|z] \setminus E[x \vee y]\}^*]$$

To show this, we compute

$$ccov(x,y) = E[E[x|z]] \vee E[E[y|z]] \setminus E[E[x|z] \vee E[y|z]]$$
$$\vee E[E[x|z] \vee E[y|z]] \setminus E[x \vee y]$$
$$= ccov(E[x|z],E[y|z]) \vee \{E[E[x|z] \vee E[y|z] - x \vee y]/E[x \vee y]^*\}$$
$$= ccov(E[x|z],E[y|z]) \vee E[ccov(x,y|z)E[x \vee y|z]^*/E[x \vee y]^*]$$

Although this is the general form, there are more useful ways of reframing it. First, observe that

$x \amalg y \mid z \Leftrightarrow ccov(x,y|z)=0$

directly from the comments made above. This condition is clearly sufficient to make the second term in the preceding equation disappear, and so we have

$ccov(x,y|z)=0 \Rightarrow ccov(x,y) = ccov(E[x|z],E[y|z])$

This is the exact parallel of

$cov(x,y|z)=0 \Rightarrow cov(x,y) = cov(E[x|z],E[y|z])$

In particular, we must have $cov(E[y|x],x|x) = ccov(E[y|x],x|x) = 0$, which establishes the parallel equations

$cov(x,y) = cov(E[y|x],x)$

$ccov(x,y) = ccov(E[y|x],x)$

We can use the latter of these equations to further substantiate the validity of the definition of ccov. Assuming that $x \longrightarrow y$ [F] and the IFR so $E[y|x] = \beta_0 \vee \beta_1 x$, we have

$ccov(x,y) = ccov(x,\beta_0 \vee \beta_1 x) = E[x] \vee E[\beta_0 \vee \beta_1 x] \setminus E[x \vee (\beta_0 \vee \beta_1 x)]$

$= E[x] \vee \beta_0 \vee \beta_1 E[x] \setminus E[\beta_0 \vee x] = \beta_1 E[x]$

This result reverberates all the way back to Section 20, reversal equation (4), which in the current context validates that the above expression is actually symmetric in x and y. It is also extremely useful for computations, since to find ccov we only need to find the conditional expectation of one factor given the other, expressed in unitary form.

Recalling that $E[y] = \beta_{0.1} \vee \beta_1 E[x]$, we now immediately have

$ccov(y,x) = P[y=1] \setminus P[y=1|x=0]$

In epidemiology the expression on the right is called the *population attributable risk*. It seems at least a little peculiar to use a measure like this, symmetric in x and y to measure the causal force of x on y. We have used β_1 here for this purpose, and it is of course not symmetric in x and y.

In the linear case, $cov(x,x) = var(x)$. In the binary case, $ccov(x,x) = E[x]$. Note the interesting fact that the regression coefficient of y on x is always $cov(x,y)/cov(x,x)$, and that in the causal model $E[y|x] = \beta_0 \vee \beta_1 x$ it is likewise true that $\beta_1 = ccov(x,y)/ccov(x,x)$.

165

Force of Causal Pathways. In classical, linear causal models there are formulas for expressing the covariance between two variables as the sum of products of coefficients, giving a decomposition of association that is due to associations along certain paths. (This is what "analysis of covariance" ought to mean, but that term has been co-opted by a different statistical procedure.) We will now turn to a simple example which suggests that the same is true for causal covariance.

We start with

$$E[y|x_1,x_2] = \beta_{0.12} \vee \beta_{1.2}x_1 \vee \beta_{2.1}x_2 \vee \beta_{12}x_1x_2$$

assumed a correctly specified model. It is immediate that

$$E[y|x_1] = \beta_{0.12} \vee \beta_{1.2}x_1 \vee (\beta_{2.1} \vee \beta_{12}x_1)(\beta_{2:0.1} \vee \beta_{2:1}x_1)$$

Now observe the general formula, where u is binary,

$$(a \vee bu)(c \vee du) = (au^* + (a \vee b)u)(cu^* + (c \vee d)u) =$$

$$= acu^* + (a \vee b)(c \vee d)u = ac \vee ((a \vee b)(c \vee d)\backslash ac)u$$

and then (using the reduction operation $u{\downarrow}v = u\backslash uv$)

$$(a \vee b)(c \vee d)\backslash ac = (a \vee b)c \vee ((a \vee b){\downarrow}c)d\backslash ac = (c{\downarrow}a)b \vee ((a \vee b){\downarrow}c)d$$

Further

$$((a \vee b){\downarrow}c)d = (a \vee b\backslash c(a \vee b))d = (a\backslash ac \vee b\backslash(c{\downarrow}a)b)d =$$

$$= (a{\downarrow}c \vee b{\downarrow}(c{\downarrow}a))d = (a{\downarrow}c)d \vee (d{\downarrow}(a{\downarrow}c))(b{\downarrow}(c{\downarrow}a))$$

Now returning to the original problem and applying these results I get

Therefore

$$ccov(y,x_1) = \{\beta_{1.2} \vee ((\beta_{2.1}{\downarrow}\beta_{2:0.1})\beta_{2:1} \vee (\beta_{2:04}{\downarrow}\beta_{2.1})\beta_{12}$$

$$\vee (\beta_{2:1}{\downarrow}(\beta_{2.1}{\downarrow}\beta_{2:0.1}))(\beta_{12}{\downarrow}(\beta_{2:04}{\downarrow}\beta_{2.1}))\}E[x_1]$$

If we now think of the causal diagram, we can envision four paths linking x_1 to y causally. In the same order as they appear above, the first goes directly from x_1 to y, and has coefficient $\beta_{1.2}$. In the second, x_1 causes x_2 which then causes y (reduced by the effect of the residual, as always). The third is where x_1 acts through the joint pathway, in conjunction with the residual of x_2 (here reduced by the direct effect). Finally, x_1 causes x_2 and then they both act through the joint pathway, reduced for effects already counted. Taken together, we have an expression for ccov(y,x_1) that provides a sensible unitary decomposition in terms of direct and indirect causal paths, despite its algebraic and conceptual complexity.

Multivariate Covariance. Conventional linear path analysis has been developed primarily within the context of the Normal distribution, in which variances and covariance summarize all there is to say about interrelationships among variables. The extension to general cases continues to assume this rather strong condition, to produce a "second order" or "weak" theory, in the language of probability theory.

It appears worthwhile to go much further with binary variables. In general, for any collection $x_1,\ldots,x_n$ of binary variables, let us define

$$\mathrm{ccov}(x_1,\ldots,x_n) = \bigvee_{i=1}^{n} E[x_i] \setminus E\left[\bigvee_{i=1}^{n} x_i\right]$$

In the case of ordinary covariance, we have formulas such as

$$\mathrm{cov}(x_1, x_2 + x_3) = \mathrm{cov}(x_1, x_2) + \mathrm{cov}(x_1, x_3)$$

In the case of causal covariance, these become

$$\mathrm{ccov}(x_1, x_2 \vee x_3) = \mathrm{ccov}(x_1, x_2, x_3) \setminus \mathrm{ccov}(x_2, x_3)$$

Or, rewritten

$$\mathrm{ccov}(x_1, x_2, x_3) = \mathrm{ccov}(x_2, x_3) \vee \mathrm{ccov}(x_1, x_2 \vee x_3)$$

suggests that the total causal covariance can be considered the covariance between any two, and the covariance of the remainder with the $\vee$-sum of those two.

Again ordinary covariance is homogeneous, in the sense that

$$\mathrm{cov}(\alpha x_1, \beta x_2) = \alpha \beta \mathrm{cov}(x_1, x_2)$$

when α, β are constants. In the causal covariance case we must put up with the more complicated

$$\mathrm{ccov}(\alpha x_1, \beta x_2) = \alpha \beta \, \mathrm{ccov}(x_1, x_2)(E[x_1 \vee x_2] \setminus E[\alpha x_1 \vee \beta x_2])*$$

167

Unitary Rates

Time plays a role in virtually all accounts of causation, if only in the dictum that causes must precede effects. I have had very little to say about time so far, and the reason is that it does not appear to be necessary to use the concept explicitly in the MSC development. Recall that in Section 10 we saw how a notion of causation denoted $\longrightarrow$ might have a core of instances of sufficient causation, denoted $\dashrightarrow$, and that if $\dashrightarrow$ were cumulative and weakly transitive, then the MSC principle extended it to a CW causation on all of $\vee\Pi F$. If the original causation were defined in terms of time, then the MSC extension would also incorporate time implicitly, even though this fact was not used in the extension process.

In this section I want to be a bit more forthcoming about how time might play a role in binary causation. The idea behind a causal equation such as

$$y = b_{0.1} \vee b_1 x_1 \qquad \text{causal}[\mathbf{F}]$$

is that it has the status of a rule that nature is required to satisfy. *Why* nature should have to do so is an intensely interesting question, but we can certainly have a very satisfactory descriptive theory of causation without yet knowing the answer. If we reflect on causal laws that might apply to continuous variables, such as movement of a physical entity, we can imagine that the rules themselves either specify or imply this continuity between cause and effect. With binary factors, however, we are deprived of continuity, because there is no way for a factor to jump from 0 to 1 continuously.

Thus, when the right side of the above causal equation becomes 1, we might expect that the left side is then required to immediately and discontinuous jump to 1 (if it were not 1 already). While there may be cases in which this describes the actual situation, surely we cannot expect such instantaneity in the crude causal fields that we actually observe. Remember in this regard Rothman's proposal that when a sufficient cause is assembled, then the disease becomes inevitable, meaning that it must happen at some indefinite future time. If we are to speak reasonably about the causes of disease that we know about, we evidently must allow for some lag in time between the instant that the right side of the causal equation becomes 1, and the later time at which the left side does.

A way to do this is to imagine that at the instant s when $b_{0,1} \lor b_1 x_1$ changes from 0 to 1 a stochastic variable T comes into existence. This variable takes values in the interval $[s, \infty]$, and is interpreted as the time that y must become 1. The probability aspect of T can be completely incorporated in its cumulative distribution function,

$$P[T \leq t\text{-}s] \quad (t \geq s)$$

We allow ∞ as a possible value only to have a formal way of saying that T never happens (that is, $T = \infty$).

We imagine that so long as $b_{0,1} \lor b_1 x_1$ remains equal to 1, we are marking time until T when y must become 1, but that if $b_{0,1} \lor b_1 x_1$ drops to 0 first, then T ceases to exist (or becomes infinite, which is the same thing). Thus, the waiting time T becomes a mathematical method of describing lags between causes and effects.

Unitary Powers. In order to cast the distribution of T into unitary terms, we require some more definitions. The first is a new operation, denoted $\diamond$ and defined for all real numbers by

$$u^{<a>} = u^{*a*}$$

We call this a *unitary power*. Note that

$$u^{<0>} = 0$$

$$u^{<1>} = u$$

The reason for the definition is

$$u^{<a>} \lor u^{<b>} = u^{*a*} \lor u^{*b*} = (u^{*a} u^{*b})^* = (u^{*(a+b)})^* = u^{<a+b>}$$

The same reasoning gives

$$u^{<a>} \lor v^{<a>} = (u \lor v)^{<a>}$$

Thus $\diamond$ behaves the same with regard to $\lor$ as ordinary powers do with respect to multiplication. For integer n, we clearly have

$$u^{<n>} = u \lor u \lor \ldots \quad (n \text{ times})$$

From

$$0 = u^{<1-1>} = u^{<1>} \vee u^{<-1>}$$

we get

$$u^{<-1>} = \backslash u$$

Compute further that

$$(u^{<a>})^{<b>} = u*^{a}**^{b}* = u*^{ab}* = u^{<ab>}$$

λn & εxp.   The function e^x or $\exp(x)$ transforms addition into multiplication

$$\exp(x+y) = \exp(x)\exp(y)$$

Correspondingly in unitary algebra, define

$$\varepsilon = 1 - e^{-1}$$

and further define the function

$$\varepsilon xp(a) = \varepsilon^{<a>}$$

It now follows immediately that εxp transforms addition into ∨,

$$\varepsilon xp(a+b) = \varepsilon xp(a) \vee \varepsilon xp(b)$$

Moreover, we can compute

$$\varepsilon xp(a) = 1 - e^{-a}$$

The inverse of $\exp(x)$ is the natural logarithm, $\ln(x)$, which transforms multiplication into addition. The corresponding unitary definition is $\lambda n(x)$ as the inverse of $\varepsilon xp(x)$, *the unitary logarithm.* Obviously

$$\lambda n(u \vee v) = \lambda n(u) + \lambda n(v)$$

and with a little work we can derive

$$\lambda n(u) = - \ln u*$$

Verify that just as $u^a = \exp(a \ln(u))$ we have $u^{<a>} = \varepsilon xp(a \lambda n(u))$.

To return to waiting times, we might posit that

$$P[T \leq t] = r^{<t>}$$

The probability density of T would then be

171

$$\frac{d}{dt} P[T \le t] = \frac{d}{dt} r^{<\triangleright} = \frac{d}{dt} r^{*t*} = \lambda n(r) \exp(-t \lambda n(r))$$

which is an exponential distribution with rate $\lambda n(r)$. We refer to r as the *unitary rate*, since it must be a unitary number in order for the cumulative distribution function of T to be increasing.

To return even further to the causal equation, a natural way to express a unitary rate in terms of the causal parameters is

$$P[T \le t | x_1] = \beta_{0.1} r_{0.1}{}^{<\triangleright} \vee \beta_1 x_1 r_1{}^{<\triangleright}$$

This model equation says two things. First, the probability that the event will ever happen is

$$P[T < \infty | x_1] = \beta_{0.1} \vee \beta_1 x_1$$

Superimposed on this eventual occurrence are rates of occurrence determined by $r_{0.1}$ and r_1. Specifically, we have two equations for the probabilitistic occurrence of T, depending on whether x_1 happens or not:

$$P[T \le t | x_1 = 0] = \beta_{0.1} r_{0.1}{}^{<\triangleright}$$

$$P[T \le t | x_1 = 1] = \beta_{0.1} r_{0.1}{}^{<\triangleright} \vee \beta_1 r_1{}^{<\triangleright}$$

This makes it explicit how the occurrence of x_1 can both raise the probability that the event will ever occur, and also increase the rate at which it will occur. For convenience these equations are expressed relative to t=0. Presumably a fully-developed theory would replace t above with the time since x_1 changed from 0 to 1.

This development can be generalized quite considerably. To do this, we need *the unitary integral*, defined by

$$\vee_0^t f(u) \mu(du) = \varepsilon xp \left(\int_0^t \lambda n(f(u)) \mu(du) \right)$$

Here μ is a measure on $[0, \infty[$, and the most familiar case would be Lebesgue measure $\mu(dt) = dt$ (the ordinary calculus integral, for all intents and purposes). The most general possible specification for a cumulative distribution function is then of the form

$$P[T \le t] = \vee_0^t r(u) \mu(du)$$

When $\mu(dt)=dt$, the function $r(t)$ is called the unitary rate function, and in the special case when it is constantly equal to r, we have

$$V_0^t \, r \, du = r^{<t>}$$

In general,

$$P[T \le t+dt] \backslash P[T \le t] = V_t^{t+dt} \, r(u)du \approx r(t)^{<dt>}$$

which is the differential version of Sheps' measure of excess occurrence.

The unitary integral appears to be the appropriate way to model waiting times arising from causal equations, because it has such natural properties in unitary algebra. For example, it is trivial to derive

$$V_0^t \, f(u)\mu(du) \vee V_0^t g(u)\mu(du) = V_0^t f(u) \vee g(u)\mu(du)$$

Moreover, if T_1 and T_2 are independent with

$$P[T_i \le t] = V_0^t \, r_i(u)\mu(du)$$

then for $T = \min\{T_1, T_2\}$ we have

$$P[T \le t] = V_0^t \, r_1(u) \vee r_2(u) \, \mu(du)$$

The importance of this result cannot be overemphasized. It says that if two stochastically independent causal process each set times T_1 and T_2 for an effect to happen, then the rate at which we observe the effect to happen is the $\vee$-sum of the individual rates. This approach (the so-called "competing risks" model) is ubiquitous in epidemiology and clinical trials methodology. One of the most interesting and difficult challenges to its use is the question of how one would come to the conclusion that two causal processes were independent of each other.

In more complex causal diagrams we can imagine that each of the causal pathways contributes to both the probability of eventual occurrence of the effect, and perhaps also to the unitary rate at which the effect happens, through $\vee$-addition of terms with individual unitary rate functions. We saw the simplest case of this above, in which the $b_{0.1}$ pathway contributed $\beta_{0.1}r_{0.1}^{<t>}$ and the b_1x_1 pathway contributed $\beta_1 x_1 r_1^{<t>}$, and implicitly the associated waiting times were independent. This provides a very satisfactory way to add some specificity to the vague notion of the "eventual occurrence" of effects.

173

Delay Times. We can flesh out the descriptive mathematics of causation in time by expanding the opportunities from ω to (t,ω), where t denotes time and ω denotes whatever kind of opportunity we were talking about before we introduced time into the picture. With this change we should say that a *factor* f is a unitary function of (t,ω) that is non-decreasing in t (and for technical reasons, we might also say that it is right-continuous in t). If there is a time t such that f(t,ω)=1 and f(t-dt,ω)=0 for all dt>0, then we say that "f happens at t". Because f cannot decrease, we are stipulating that a factor indicates an event that can happen at most once. It is always possible to take into account a series of "identical" events, by labeling them as the first, the second, the third, and so on, and clearly a "first event" can happen at most once.

A *delay time* is a binary function of the form $\tau(u{:}s,\omega)$. The *convolution* of a delay time with a factor f is

$$\tau{\bullet}f(t) = \int_0^t \tau(t - u{:}u)df(u)$$

Because f jumps at most at one time point, the measure df(u) is really just an evaluation at the jump point. Thus, if f happens at s and the factor $\tau(t{:}s)$ happens at t=u, then $\tau{\bullet}f$ happens at s+u.

Now the way I want to use this is to think of x as a factor that has some intrinsic meaning, and τ as a factor that will delay the effect of x, so that τ•x is the delayed time at which x will have an effect. This is how I am going to deal with "eventual occurrence".

With factors defined as above, we must re-define non-trivial implication. f $\xrightarrow{\text{NT}}$ y means there exists a τ for which $0 \neq \tau{\bullet}f \leq y$. This means that y can happen no later than τ•f. Once f happens, we know there is a later time by which y must have happened. If τ=1 identically, then τ•f =f and we have immediate implication. Recall that for a sufficient causation we now have

f $\xrightarrow{\text{s}}$ y ⇒ there exists a τ such that $0 \neq \tau{\bullet}f \leq y$

This says that if f happens, then there is some definite time afterwards that y must have happened, specifically the time that τ•f happens.

We would then require that $\xrightarrow{\text{s}}$ is weakly transitive (W) and cumulative (C). Therefore, if we were to start with $\xrightarrow{\text{s}}$ defined on a

174

specific collection **F** of factors, then we could extend it to a sufficient CW causation on $\lor\Pi\mathbf{F}$.

This provides a compact way to write structural causal equations. If we have a general expression like

$$C[y|\mathbf{F}] = \lor\{b_A x_A : A \subseteq N\} \qquad \text{causal}[\mathbf{F}]$$

then since each pathway $b_A x_A$ is a sufficient cause of y, there must exist a corresponding delay time τ_A, and so if all of the causes of y lie in **F**, then we can write

$$y = \lor\{\tau_A \bullet (b_A x_A) : A \subseteq N\} \qquad \text{causal}[\mathbf{F}]$$

(When not all the causes are in **F**, then the right side will consist of only part of y, the part caused by factors in **F**.) Note the intriguing possibility that if one of the factors $\tau_A \bullet (b_A x_A)$ happens first, then we might say that is *the singular* cause of y *in this situation*. In the case of ties, there would still be attributional ambiguity.

The material in this section does not exhaust the problems that accompany any attempt to incorporate time into the MSC framework. There remains a substantial amount of work to describe temporal aspects of MSC systems adequately. These lead to the fundamental question of how contradictory causal equations are adjudicated, a topic that must remain for another time.

Functional Causation

One of the most natural definitions of causation involves functional relations, such as

$$y = fctn(x)$$

Here, I am going to use the "fctn" notation as a template, just as I used pr(x) and pr(y|x) earlier (see Section 4). This will let me write about functional relationships easily, plugging in specific functions when I need to.

So the essential part of the above equation is that for each x there is a corresponding y, and the "fctn" is simply a rule that tells how to find the y, given the x. From this description, it should be clear that the mathematical purpose of a function is to encode information. It seems reasonable to say that both x and the function carry information about y, because x together with the definition of the function gives me y.

We might be willing to say that instances of our notion of causation imply functional relationships If we were to take nontrivial implication as an example, when I write

$$C[y|F] = y = b_{0.1} \lor b_1 x_1 \qquad\qquad \text{causal}[F]$$

surely this implies that

$$y = fctn(x_1, b_{0.1}, b_1)$$

It is important in this case to see that the functional equation does not serve as a definition of causation. The causal equation, with its residual cause and co-cause, as defined within the causal field, specify NI as a causation. The functional relationship is an off-shoot of the causal definition. Nevertheless, one might take this example to mean that a definition of cause could be constructed out of a functional relationship, plus something else.

Rubin's HRP is an example. Recall from Section 28 that in this theory each instance ω is associated with two factors, $\eta(0, \omega)$ and $\eta(1, \omega)$, and the assumption is that $y = \eta(x(\omega), \omega)$, a functional relationship. Note the very important fact, however, that this is not a relationship of the form $y = fctn(x)$. This latter equation would say that the value of x alone is sufficient to determine y, but Rubin's HRP also allows us to use the value of ω for the specific instance as well. This means that in the HRP system, y can depend functionally on anything that can be determined from ω, which includes, of course $f(\omega)$ for all f in **F**. It was precisely this fact that made difficulties in Section 28, since changing x could cause changes in the f's, which could violate pre-existing causal laws, and which had an impact on the defined value of y. The purpose of this section is to examine an alternative approach to this problem.

Another reason that a functional relation cannot serve as a definition of causation is that often functions are reversible, but the causal process is not. For example, in an individual whose general health (and in particular the state of his heart muscle) does not change over a period of time, systolic blood pressure is a function of vascular resistance, and this is a causal relation. (Vascular resistance is increased by narrowing of the blood vessels, usually through an atherosclerotic process, and by loss of tone - the ability to constrict or dilate - of the blood vessel walls.) As the person's vascular resistance increases, so does the systolic blood pressure, and this happens in a strictly increasing fashion. This means that for any particular systolic blood pressure, we can find the corresponding vascular resistance (so $x = fctn(y)$), but certainly this does not mean that systolic blood pressure causes narrowing of the arteries.

Pearl & Verma's Definition. In a long series of articles (initiated by reference 1), Judea Pearl and his colleagues have posed a causal definition in the form

$$y = g(x,e) \qquad\qquad e \amalg x$$

Here e is defined on Ω, and so with our random sampling probability P, it is a random variable. There is no restriction on it, however, so it could take values in an arbitrary (measurable) space. x, on the other hand, is a factor, taking values in $\{0,1\}$. It is an essential part of the definition that e be independent of x, and we will see that this has some considerable consequences.

The first consequence is that Pearl's approach is counterfactual. This is because in order for x and e to be independent, neither can restrict the possible values of the other. In particular, the fact that $e(\omega)$ assumes some value cannot restrict $x(\omega)$ to being 0, and likewise cannot restrict it to being 1. This means that x can assume either of its values at any opportunity, which was also a fundamental assumption of Rubin's hypothetical response profile (HRP). For this reason, we can refer to $g(0,e)$ and $g(1,e)$ as Pearl's HRP.

In fact, it is convenient to define $a_0 = g(0,e)$ and $a_1 = g(1,e)$ as factors defined on Ω. Since $y = a_0 x^* \vee a_1 x$, it is clear that these two factors summarize everything about e that is useful for knowing y. By assuming that $a_0 \amalg x$ and $a_1 \amalg x$, this definition tries to deal with the problems caused by counterfactual reasoning.

To fit this into the MSC framework, it seems reasonable to take $F = \{x, x^*, a_0, a_1\}$. Thus we see that the first distinction between MSC and Pearl's approach is that in MSC we start out with the factors F defined from some set of considerations, but in Pearl's approach we acquire them as part of the definition. The second distinction is that MSC does not use any probability distribution on Ω, whereas Pearl's approach absolutely requires it. I introduced P as random sampling in Section 8 merely to provide an empirical link between observations we can make, and the population from which those observations came. There are, of course, other probability distributions than random sampling. This does not disturb MSC theory, because it does not depend on P. It does mean, however, that Pearl's theory depends on P. This has the consequence that every method of sampling the population provides its own causal theory, and these need not agree for the fixed collection of variables in which we are interested. Although troubling, these issues lead us far from where I want to go, and so for present purposes I assume that random sampling P is the appropriate definition for Pearl's theory.

Before going on, I should also say that Pearl and his colleagues do not seem to actually say that "$y = g(x,e)$ with $e \amalg x$" defines causation. Instead, they employ this condition in situations where they talk about "causal models", "causal theories", or "causal hypotheses". I would imagine that this is a rhetorical device to avoid being castigated by those who have been brain-damaged by Hume's skepticism, but in any case, I do not feel that I am stretching their intent by taking their condition as a definition.

It seems clear that as I have presented it here, Pearl's theory is a particular case of nontrivial implication. That is, in the absence of a discussion of time, we should take $g(x,e)=1$ to mean that the eventual occurrence of y is assured. I will not try to solve the problems of accounting for time here, because I don't think they are necessary in order to contrast MSC and Pearl's approach.

Applying the MSC method to the definition gives

$$y = a_0 a_1 \lor a_0 x^* \lor a_1 x \qquad \text{causal}[\mathbf{F}]$$

This is an example of paradoxical causation (Section 27). This arises because in Pearl's general theory y and x are not restricted to being factors, so that the sense of covariation need not be specified. We should note that even though this is paradoxical causation, with the independence assumptions in force here, causal effect parameters are identifiable. It seems that this specialization of Pearl's theory would come closer to our usual idea of causation for factors, however, if we were to assume that $a_0 x \xrightarrow{\text{NI}} a_1 x$, because we would then have

$$y = a_0 \lor a_1 x \qquad \text{causal}[\mathbf{F}]$$

In this specialization, we again have as a fundamental assumption that a_0 $\amalg$ x, which is the IFR. This points up yet another distinction between MSC and Pearl's HRP. Whereas MSC permits model miss-specification in the presence of genuine causation, the HRP approach takes it as part of the definition that such miss-specification does not happen.

This goes back to a point that was made in Section 19. There I indicated that it was possible for x_1 to cause y only through its causation of x_2 (an indirect causal chain), where this did not imply that y $\amalg$ $x_1|x_2$ *unless the model was correctly specified.* Any theory that takes correct model specification as part of its definition of causation will have the theorem "indirect causation $\Rightarrow$ conditional independence", but this is not an MSC theorem.

To finish this set of ideas, under the assumptions of Pearl's HRP (and our specialization) it follows immediately that $\beta_{0.1} = E[a_0]$ and $\beta_1 = E[a_1] \setminus E[a_0]$.

Much of the work of Pearl and colleagues is to examine more complex situations than the one I inspected here. This research is enormously useful for studying systems of interrelated variables, and one may perhaps overlook the fact that at least some of the relative simplicity of their theory is a consequence of the rather strong conditions they place on their basic definition of causation. As an example of this, consider Figure 1. The fundamental conditions intended here are $x_3 \amalg x_4|x_5$, $(x_1,x_2) \amalg x_5|(x_3,x_4)$, and $x_1 \amalg x_2|(x_3,x_4)$. These are implied by the assumption of the functional conditions

$$x_1 = f_1(x_3,x_4,e_1)$$

$$x_2 = f_2(x_3,x_4,e_2)$$

$$x_3 = f_3(x_5,e_3)$$

$$x_4 = f_4(x_5,e_4)$$

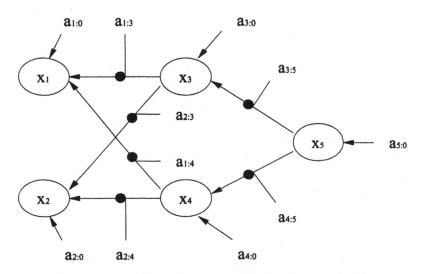

Figure 1. With the functional definition of causation, there are no relationships between x's and a's that would result in a mis-specified model.

where the e's are independent of each other and independent of the x's with which they are paired in parentheses. From this strong assumption, we can define all the a's of Figure 1 just as we did in the simple case of two factors. The important point is that it follows as a consequence of the functional conditions and the independence assumptions that the IFR, and the CIFC hold in all causal equations. All miss-specification problems except those associated with CICC disappear as a matter of definition. It is, therefore, not possible to talk about functional causation and model miss-specification in the same breath; the two ideas are mutually incompatible, by definition. If I had included joint pathways in Figure 1, then by the failure of CICC they might have been miss-specified.

Regression Futility. Let me finish this section with a completely different functional theory, which fails miserably. It is a fact that

$$y = h(x) + \varepsilon$$

with $E[\varepsilon] = 0$ and $cov(x,\varepsilon)=0$. In fact, $h(x)$ is $E[y|x]$. (This result is true of more general y and x, with the sole change that ε is uncorrelated with any function of x.) In the case of factors, this is the same as linear regression, because every function of a factor is linear. The idea is that if $h(0) \neq h(1)$, then $y = fctn(x,\varepsilon)$ depends genuinely on x, and that ε is perhaps not quite independent of x, but close to being independent, and so x should be a cause of y. One problem with this is that it would show that virtually every factor is a cause of every other, a situation that offends even our commonsense notion of cause. The second problem is that if we assume that h does not take the values 0 or 1 (the usual case), then y is the indicator of $[\varepsilon>0]$. That is, $y = fctn(\varepsilon)$ which seems to vitiate the previous argument that y genuinely depended on x. This suggests that conditional expectation and regression models cannot serve as definitions of causation without supplemental considerations.

Reference

1. Pearl J, Verma TS. A theory of inferred causation. In JA Allen, R Fikes, and E. Sandwell (Eds.) *Principles of Knowledge Representation and Reasoning: Proceeding of the Second International Congress.* San Mateo CA: Morgan Kaufmann, pp. 441-452, 1991

The Causation Operator

In this section I want to develop some of the properties of the sufficient cause operator, $C[y|F]$. This operator was defined in Section 6. There I assumed that $\longrightarrow$ was an MSC causation, which meant that it was cumulative (C) and weakly transitive (W), and that it had a nonempty core of sufficient causal relations (denoted $\overset{s}{\longrightarrow}$) which was also CW. It followed that $\overset{s}{\longrightarrow}$ is transitive (T), and that it can be extended consistently to be a CSW (and therefore T) causation on all of $\vee\Pi F$. The sufficient cause of y in F was then defined as

$$C[y|F] = \vee\{f \in \Pi F : f \overset{s}{\longrightarrow} y\}$$

The important facts about $C[y|F]$ are

$$C[y|F] \overset{s}{\longrightarrow} y$$

$$C[y|F] \leq y$$

For $f \in \vee\Pi F$, $f \overset{s}{\longrightarrow} C[y|F] \Leftrightarrow f \overset{nt}{\longrightarrow} C[y|F] \Leftrightarrow f \overset{s}{\longrightarrow} y$

The properties that we will establish for $C[y|F]$ are motivated by wanting it to behave like the conditional expectation operator, $E[y|F]$.

Here is the first property:

$$y_1 \overset{s}{\longrightarrow} y_2 \Rightarrow C[y_1|F] \leq C[y_2|F] \qquad \text{(Left Monotone)}$$

By transitivity, $f \overset{s}{\longrightarrow} y_1 \overset{s}{\longrightarrow} y_2$ implies $f \overset{s}{\longrightarrow} y_2$, completing the demonstration. This implication is not generally reversible. Note, however, that the right side implies $C[y_1|F] \overset{s}{\longrightarrow} y_2$, and this would yield the left side in the special case $y_1 = C[y_1|F]$.

The corresponding property involves restricting the factors under consideration

$$G \subseteq F \Rightarrow C[y|G] \leq C[y|F] \qquad \text{(Right Monotone)}$$

which follows from the observation that for $g \in \Pi G$, $g \overset{s}{\longrightarrow} y$ implies $g \overset{nt}{\longrightarrow} C[y|F]$.

The next property justifies calling $C[y|F]$ a projection operator:

$$G \subseteq F \Rightarrow C[y|G] = C[C[y|F]|G] \qquad \text{(Smoothing Equation)}$$

Since $C[y|F] \xrightarrow{s} y$, we have $C[C[y|F]|G] \leq C[y|G]$ by left monotonicity. On the other hand, for $g \in \Pi G$, $g \xrightarrow{s} y$ implies $g \xrightarrow{s} C[y|F]$, which implies $C[y|G] \leq C[C[y|F]|G]$, completing the demonstration.

Regular Causations. There are many properties of the sufficient cause operator that can be demonstrated under special conditions. A set of assumptions that is particularly useful are those under which $\xrightarrow{s}$ is *regular* (R):

(R$_1$) $f_1 \xrightarrow{s} y_1$, $f_2 \xrightarrow{s} y_2$ $(f_1, f_2 \in \vee \Pi F) \Rightarrow f_1 \vee f_2 \xrightarrow{s} y_1 \vee y_2$

(R$_2$) $f_1 \xrightarrow{s} y_1$, $f_2 \xrightarrow{s} y_2$, $f_1 f_2 \neq 0$ $(f_1, f_2 \in \vee \Pi F) \Rightarrow f_1 f_2 \xrightarrow{s} y_1 y_2$

(R$_3$) $f \xrightarrow{s} y$, $fg \neq 0 \Rightarrow gf \xrightarrow{s} gy$

These are reasonable conditions for a sufficient causation to satisfy, and it is easy to check that they hold for nontrivial implication. R_1 would be argued by saying that if our notion of sufficient causation involved the notion of "production" of the effect, as many theories do, then if f_1 produces y_1 and f_2 produces y_2, then knowing that one of f_1 or f_2 happened certainly means that one of y_1 or y_2 will be produced. Likewise, R_2 says that if we know they both happened, then both of the effects they produce happen. R_3 is a little less straightforward, because it in effect says that sufficient causes with respect to Ω remain sufficient causes when we restrict consideration to a proper subset $[g=1]$.

The main result of this section is then

If $\xrightarrow{s}$ is R, then

$$C[y_1|F]\, C[y_2|F] = C[y_1 y_2|F]$$

$$C[y_1|F] \vee C[y_2|F] = C[y_1 \vee y_2|F]$$

$$C[fy|F] = f\, C[y|F] \quad (f \in \vee \Pi F)$$

For the first equation, proving $(\leq)$ is easy, since $f_i \leq C[y_i|F]$ implies $f_i \xrightarrow{s} y_i$ which implies $f_1 f_2 \xrightarrow{s} y_1 y_2$ (or $f_1 f_2 = 0$) so that $f_1 f_2 \leq C[y_1 y_2|F]$. To prove $(\geq)$, let $f \xrightarrow{s} y_1 y_2$ and $g \xrightarrow{s} y_1$. Now $f \xrightarrow{NI} f \vee g \xrightarrow{s} y_1 y_2 \vee y_1 = y_1$

184

shows $f \overset{\blacksquare}{\longrightarrow} y_1$, and a similar argument shows $f \overset{\blacksquare}{\longrightarrow} y_2$, so that $f \leq$ $C[y_1|F]C[y_2|F]$. This demonstrates the first equation.

For the second equation, ($\leq$) follows directly from R_1. For ($\geq$), let $f \overset{\blacksquare}{\longrightarrow} y_1 \vee y_2$. This implies $f = fy_1 \vee fy_2$. By R_3, each fy_i is either 0 or else $fy_i \overset{\blacksquare}{\longrightarrow} (y_1 \vee y_2)y_i = y_i$, which shows $fy_1 \vee fy_2 \leq C[y_1|F] \vee C[y_2|F]$. This completes the proof of the second equation.

For the third equation, $C[fy|F] = C[f|F]C[y|F] \leq f\,C[y|F]$. Conversely, since $C[y|F] \overset{\blacksquare}{\longrightarrow} y$ by R_3 we have $fC[y|F] \overset{\blacksquare}{\longrightarrow} fy$ so that $fC[y|F] \leq$ $C[fy|F]$. This completes the demonstration.

Remarks on C. Distinguishing $C[y|F]$ from y itself seems to be a step forward in even talking about causation. Many theories try to relate effect y to its causes $\{x_i\}$ without the intermediary of $C[y|F]$. This creates special difficulties when there is delay in causation, as there must be most of the time. Once $C[y|F]$ happens, then except for the possibility of new causal instances in the future, y will happen, and the underlying process is causal. As we have seen, substituting "cause of $C[y|F]$" for "cause of y" would amount to remarkably little change, at least for CSW causations and the MSC causations they generate. From the practical standpoint, however, it is y that is named and measured, while $C[y|F]$ most often goes unnoticed, and is perhaps not capable of being noticed.

Causal Modeling

The purpose of modeling is usually to try to say something about all the causal influences among a collection of variables. This inevitably leads to some assumptions that would justify the modeling process. As we have seen, to reason about causal relationships a fairly daunting number of assumptions appear to be required. In this section we blithely assume them all, in order to see what the modeling consequences would be.

Without the blithe assumptions, we have the structural equation

$$y = \vee \{b_A x_A : A \subseteq N\} \qquad \text{causal[F]}$$

where $N = \{1,\dots,n\}$, and with them we get the notationally satisfying

$$E[y|x_1,\dots,x_n] = \vee\{\beta_A x_A : A \subseteq N\}$$

Recall that with this notation $x_A = \Pi\{x_i : i \in A\}$. We call this the *unitary statistical model*.

Another way of expressing this is

$$\lambda n(E[y|x_1,\dots,x_n]) = \Sigma\{\alpha_A x_A: A \subseteq N\}$$

where $\alpha_A = \lambda n(\beta_A)$. In statistical jargon, this is a *generalized linear model*, with λn as the *link* function. For our purposes, I will call this a *complementary exponential model*. Many statistical packages have routines for fitting this kind of model. This shows that with the powerful assumptions that are necessary for correct specification of a multi-factor causal model, the statistical problems have already been solved.

Unitary Explanatory Variables. I now want to widen the modeling sphere, by considering arbitrary unitary variables denoted $z_1,\dots,z_n$. This generalizes the situation I have just been discussing, since factors are special cases of unitary variables, and so some of the z's could be x's , and others could be products of x's. But by allowing the z's to be unitary, I allow intermediate values between zero and one, and this is the point of the generalization.

For a factor x, it is clear that $\beta x = \beta^{<x>} = \exp(\alpha x)$ where $\alpha = \lambda n(\beta)$. Consequently, a sensible way to extend the causal model to unitary factors like the z's is with the complementary exponential model

$$\lambda n(E[y|z_1,\ldots,z_n]) = \Sigma\{\alpha_i z_i : i = 1,\ldots,n\}$$

It is not true for unitary z that $\beta z = \beta^{<z>}$, so this proposal represents a selection between the model above and the unitary statistical model

$$E[y|z_1,\ldots,z_n] = \vee\{\beta_i z_i : i=1,\ldots,n\}$$

In the absence of a more fully developed theory for unitary factors, there is no way to choose between these, and since the former can be fitted by existing statistical software whereas the latter cannot, there is some, perhaps transient, practical reason to favor the complementary exponential model.

In all situations up to this point, the effect has been a factor, but now I want to include more general effect measures. I will revert to standard statistical notation by letting Y stand for an outcome measurement, defined on a scale so that the event that Y exceeds a specific value y, [Y>y], is well defined. In particular, Y could be a measurement made on the real number line, but that is not the only case covered here. Similarly, I will temporarily use X for the cause, taking values x. The unitary statistical model then becomes

$$P[Y>y|X=x] = \beta_0(y)\vee\beta_1(y)x$$

In general, the β-parameters could also depend on x, but this leads to more complications than I want to deal with at the moment. Note that if X is a factor, then for each y this is the kind of model we have seen a great deal. Otherwise, X should be rescaled to take values between 0 and 1, so that it is a unitary variable. There are a number of practical ways of carrying out such a transformation, perhaps the easiest being to replace X with (X-Min)/(Max-Min), where Min and Max are the effective minimum and maximum value that X can assume.

188

If we integrate both sides of the above model equation with respect to pr(dx|X>x), which is the conditional distribution of X given that X>x, then we get

$$P[Y>y|X>x] = \beta_0(y) \vee \beta_1(y)\, E[X|X>x]$$

Note that this reduces our original observations to two factors, one for [Y>y] and one for [X>x], but that the above model is a little different than the unitary statistical model for factors, due to the replacement of the indicator of [X>x] on the right with the expected value of X for values of X above x.

Suppose now that Y is also unitary (or transformed so as to make it unitary). If we assume β_1 free of y, then we have the *constant causal effect model*. Integrating with respect to dy over [0,1], in the original unitary model equation, we get

$$E[Y|X=x] = \beta_0 \vee \beta_1 x$$

where

$$\beta_0 = \int_0^1 \beta_0(y)\,dy$$

This model is, of course, different than the usual linear regression model that is used in these cases. It is extremely attractive for use in general causal diagrams, though.

I have developed these models with only one cause, but it is clear that they can easily be extended. For general unitary Z_i we would start with

$$P[Y>y|Z_1=z_1,\ldots,Z_k=z_k] = \beta_0(y) \vee \beta_1(y)z_1 \vee \ldots \vee \beta_k(y)z_k$$

Following the same steps as above, we get to

$$E[Y|Z_1,\ldots,Z_k] = \beta_0 \vee \beta_1 Z_1 \vee \ldots \vee \beta_k Z_k$$

Prospection & Retrospection. There is a variety of statistical approaches to estimate the β or α parameters and perform inference on them, but the one I would like to concentrate on here is likelihood inference in the case where the effect is a factor and the causes are unitary:

189

$$P[Y=1|z_1,\ldots,z_k] = \beta_0 \vee \beta_1 z_1 \vee \ldots \beta_k z_k$$

for the unitary statistical model, and

$$P[Y=1|z_1,\ldots,z_k] = \exp(\alpha_0 + \alpha_1 z_1 + \ldots + \alpha_k z_k)$$

for the complementary exponential model. It will turn out that the only function I need to deal with is

$$R(z) = \frac{P\big[Y=1|z\big]}{P\big[Y=0|z\big]}$$

where I have used z to abbreviate $(z_1,\ldots,z_k)$, and I have also suppressed the dependence on the parameters, so they could be either the β's or the α's. I will elaborate on this in a moment, but first it is useful to distinguish the prospective and retrospective observation designs.

In the prospective design I study a collection of individuals with z-values that I regard as being fixed numbers. Even though I might have sampled people from some population, I nonetheless regard their z-values as fixed, and not as the result of some sampling procedure. In this case, R(z) is sufficient for doing inference, because

$$P[Y=1|z] = R(z)/(1+R(z))$$

so I can calculate the likelihood from the Y-observations and the corresponding values of R(z) (as we will see in a moment).

In the retrospective design it is a little more complex. Here I acquire a sample from the population [Y=1] and another sample from the population [Y=0], and then I look on the corresponding z-values as random variables - that is, as having been produced by a sampling process. In this situation, the only ingredients for doing inference are pr′(z|Y=1) and pr′(z|Y=0), the conditional distributions of the z's given the value of Y. I put primes on these to emphasize that they pertain to the retrospective design. The question I want to answer is, how can I turn this around to do inference about the β's (or the α's)?

The answer is through the reversal equations, expressed now as

$$P'[Y=1|z]\ pr'(z) = pr'(z|Y=1)P'[Y=1]$$

Note that this mixes the template notation (pr) with the probability notation P, because I know Y is a factor, but z could consist of factors, or of unitary variables with continuous distributions, or mixtures, so I want to include all these cases in one argument. (That is why the template notation is useful.) The other reversal equation is

$$P'[Y=0|z]pr'(z) = pr'(z|Y=0)P'[Y=0]$$

Here is where the argument gets a little slippery, so we have to be very careful what we mean. First, in the retrospective design I either know $P'[Y=1]$, or I'm willing to regard it as known, so that it gives me no information about the parameters. In practice, this means that I set $P'[Y=1]$ equal to the fraction of $[Y=1]$ cases in my data. Secondly, I assume that $pr'(z)$ contains no useful information about the parameters. This is essentially the same as assuming that all of the information about the parameters is in $pr'(z|Y=y)$ for $y=0,1$. Under these two assumptions, the values $pr'(z|Y=y)$ are sufficient for computing the likelihood, and this is the same as saying (under the two assumptions) that the values $P'[Y=y|z]$ are sufficient for computing the same likelihood. So far, my assumptions have given me the result that I can do inference from the likelihood based on $pr'(z|Y=y)$ or from $P'[Y=y|z]$, and the choice is mine. I make the second choice, because that will make the retrospective analysis look more like the prospective analysis.

But this choice leads to one further complexity, that I now resolve. Going back to the prospective study, I can also write down the reversal equations

$$P[Y=1|z]pr(z) = pr(z|Y=1)P[Y=1]$$

$$P[Y=0|z]pr(z) = pr(z|Y=0)P[Y=0]$$

There are no primes on these, because they are the prospective probabilities. It is important to realize that the retrospective probabilities (with primes) can be different from the prospective probabilities (without primes). The fundamental assumption that connects prospective with retrospective studies is that

$$pr(z|Y=y) = pr'(z|Y=y)$$

This means that even though the two designs obtained people in different ways, the implied conditional distributions of causes z given effect outcomes Y are the same. I pause only for an instant to point out that trying to make this assumption plausible is the central difficulty of retrospective studies in epidemiology.

The key equation is now

$$R(z) = \frac{P[Y = 1|z]}{P[Y = 0|z]} = \frac{pr(z|Y = 1)P[Y = 1]}{pr(z|Y = 0)P[Y = 0]} =$$

$$= \frac{pr'(z|Y = 1)P'[Y = 1]}{pr'(z|Y = 0)P'[Y = 0]}\rho = \frac{P'[Y = 1|z]}{P'[Y = 0|z]}\rho = R'(z)\rho$$

where

$$\rho = \frac{P[Y = 1]P'[Y = 0]}{P[Y = 0]P'[Y = 1]}$$

Recall that I said above that in the retrospective design, I was willing to use $R'(z)$ to construct the likelihood. I explicitly made two model assumptions that justified this. The problem that I am now trying to solve is that the parameters I am interested in (β's or α's) are naturally expressed in $R(z)$, but not so easily in $R'(z)$. The key equation above has established a relationship between these two, and this resolves the problem. In the retrospective design

P'[Y=1|z] = R'(z)/(1+R'(z)) = R(z)/(ρ+R(z))

Therefore, I can construct the appropriate likelihood in the retrospective design from the R(z) function of the prospective design, provided only that I know ρ.

I pointed out that in the retrospective design P'[Y=1] is set equal to the fraction of [Y=1] in the study, which is a value set by the investigators (usually ½, but not always). The only other piece of information required for ρ is P[Y=1], which is usually interpreted as the prevalence of the disease in the population.

The slippery argument is now over, so it is time to sum up. In either a retrospective or prospective study, with a collection z of causes and factor Y as effect, the likelihood for the parameters can be constructed from

$$P[Y = 1|z] = \frac{R(z)}{\rho + R(z)}$$

where $\rho=1$ in the prospective design, and is given by the equation three paragraphs back in the retrospective design. As a consequence, all likelihood inference can be based on the above equation with ρ known.

Likelihood Inference. The remainder of this section assumes an understanding of likelihood inference, and the reader who does not have this preparation is encouraged to acquire it before proceeding.

The log likelihood is now of the form

$$\ell = \sum y \ln R(z) - \ln(\rho + R(z))$$

Here the summation is over all individuals in the study, but all subscripts are suppressed. y is the indicator of the effect, and z is the vector of causes. In what follows, I let **D** stand for the column vector of derivatives with respect to the parameters (β's or α's).

Compute

$$\mathbf{D}\ell = \sum y\mathbf{D} \ln R(z) - \mathbf{D} \ln(\rho + R(z)) = \sum \left(y - \frac{R(z)}{\rho + R(z)} \right)\mathbf{D} \ln R(z) \text{ As}$$

usual, the maximum likelihood estimates are found by solving

$$\mathbf{D}\ell = \mathbf{0}$$

The other quantity needed for a likelihood inference is the negative second derivative of the log likelihood. In order to reduce variability in this quantity, its expectation is usually computed (here it would be the conditional expectation of the y's given the z's). After some algebra, this reduces to

$$E[-\mathbf{D}\mathbf{D}'\ell] = \sum \frac{\rho R(z)}{(\rho + R(z))^2}\mathbf{D} \ln R(z)\mathbf{D}' \ln R(z)$$

The two cases of interest here would be the unitary and complementary exponential models. The unitary statistical model is the more complex of the two, since

$$R(z) = \frac{\beta_0 \vee \bigvee_{i=1}^{k} \beta_i z_i}{\beta_0^* \prod_{i=1}^{k} (\beta_i z_i)^*}$$

The complementary exponential model is just

$$R(z) = \frac{\exp\left(\alpha_0 + \sum_{i=1}^{k} \alpha_i z_i\right)}{\exp\left(\alpha_0 + \sum_{i=1}^{k} \alpha_i z_i\right)^*} = \exp\left(\alpha_0 + \sum_{i=1}^{k} \alpha_i z_i\right) - 1$$

again showing that the computationally easiest case (the complementary exponential) may not be the most intellectually satisfying case (the unitary statistical model).

This finishes the remarks that I want to make about inference in the prospective and retrospective designs. I cannot resist pointing out, however, that if one adopts the logistic model

$$P[Y=1|z] = \exp(\beta_0+\beta'z)/(1+\exp(\beta_0+\beta'z))$$

then

$$R(z) = \exp(\beta_0+\beta'z)$$

and this choice simplifies the computational problem quite considerably. Although it may not be obvious, the only difference between prospective and retrospective inference (in the logistic case) is in the β_0 term. This means that one can analyze retrospective data exactly as if it were prospective data, so long as one ignores the β_0 term. The attractiveness of this computational accident has so entranced epidemiologists that they have embraced the logistic model (with its odds ratio association measure) to the exclusion of all other models.

The point of view that I take here is that mathematical beauty is in the eye of the mathematical beholder. It may be that nature has arranged things so that our conception of mathematical harmony corresponds to the realities that she dictates, or maybe not. I tend to think that a more fundamental analysis, such as that based on the MSC approach, will lead us to how nature actually works, and whether we regard the resulting mathematics and computation as pretty or ugly is irrelevant.

Causes of Teenage Smoking. I finish this relatively long section with an example. The data here were collected from 200 tenth and eleventh-grade girls. The key issue of the study was to account for the trial or

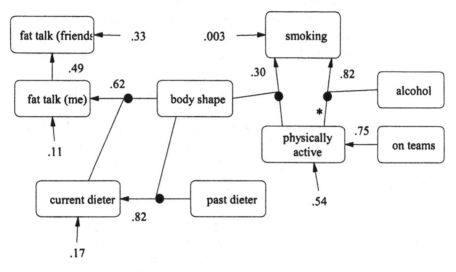

Figure 1. A causal diagram oriented toward finding the causes of smoking.

adoption of smoking cigarettes, which about one in four girls will have done. One theory was that concern about *body shape* together with the belief that smoking causes thinness (*thinness*) would cause smoking. A large number of other variables were measured, and in addition to the two just mentioned, the remainder appear in Figure 1.

Smoking was a factor, but all the other variables were unitary, having been transformed from Likert scales to the 0-1 scale. The models were all of the form given above, with $\lambda n(E[y|z])$ linear in the z's. The coefficients shown in Figure 1 are β's (not α's). Note that each β is the exp of its corresponding α.

195

The Figure was produced by fitting a very large number of different models, and retaining only those with impressively statistically and practically significant parameters. Subject-matter knowledge was also used to determine the directions of some of the arrows. It was the intent that those arrows not appearing in Figure 1, that might have been there, were tested and are actually absent in reality. There is at this time no program that automatically searches for good models of this form.

Some of the causal relationships were not surprises. That participation *on teams* causes higher *physical activity* is almost a tautology. It is perhaps not a surprise that *past dieting* behavior together with concern about *body shape* caused *current dieting*, but it was a bit of a surprise that both factors were in the pathway, and that there were no pathways involving either factor without the other. (Past dieting was actually measured in the past, removing perhaps some of the potential artifactual association between dietary reports taken at the same time.) Similarly, *body shape* and *current dieting* appeared to both be necessary in causing the girl to engage in "fat talk" about herself (*fat talk (me)*). Willingness to engage in such talk in social situations (*fat talk(friends)*) was caused only by *fat talk(me)* and not by concern with *body shape*.

The largest surprise is that virtually all of the *smoking* behavior can be accounted for (residual cause only .003). The two dominant pathways are first, a strong one involving *alcohol* use and low *physical activity*. The other pathway involved *body shape* and *physical activity*. This suggests two pathways to smoking, one involving sedentarism and alcohol consumption, and the other involving concern about body shape, but only when accompanied with physical activity. Note that causation is paradoxical with regard to *physical activity*.

Perhaps the most unconventional finding of this study was that belief that smoking keeps you thin (*thinness*) never appeared to be associated with any other factor (no less smoking), and it never participated in any pathway causing smoking, which is why it doesn't appear in Figure 1. Secondly, while it is conventional to imagine that concern with *body shape* will be a cause of dieting, why physical activity should be a co-cause of *body shape* in causing smoking requires further explanation.

Construction of Figure 1 is only part of a causal analysis. Another important part is interpretation, since there is nothing in the mathematics of statistical estimation that guarantees the capture of causal relationships alone. In some cases this is easy. Girls who have dieted in the past and who are concerned about their body shape naturally continue to diet. It is also natural to imagine that the girls who diet and worry about their bodies will engage in conversation about these issues. In other cases interpretation is more problematic. One could certainly argue that there is nothing inherent in alcohol consumption (either with or without physical activity) that would lead to smoking. Both could move together simply due to maturation - but this is ruled out by the fact that grade in school (indicator of 11th graders) was not associated with smoking or alcohol in any detectable fashion. In fact, a better alternative explanation would be that both drinking and smoking were part of a syndrome of experimentation with adult behaviors that are illegal for teenagers (at least in the United States), and that perhaps low physical activity is a surrogate for individuals who have that syndrome. We cannot expect the causal analysis to uncover this from the data available, since there were no items that had been designed to capture a propensity for experimentation, but surely it is a virtue of the causal analysis that it turned up the need for such an item.

In summary, this section has collected a large number of threads spun in earlier sections. Structural causal models for binary variables (factors) can be plausibly extended to cases in which causes and effects are measured on ordinal scales. Every structural model implies a probability model, under enough simplifying assumptions. When a transformation to the unitary scale is possible, then existing statistical software is available for prospective analyses. A simple modification of the prospective computational routines solves the problem of retrospective designs. In a smoking example, we have seen that it is possible to sit down with the tools that have been discussed, and reason with the data about potential causal relationships, using statistical and practical criteria for assessing strength of association and our personal notion of causation as a guide to structure and interpretation.

Dependence

It is not uncommon to see a notion of causation expressed in terms of "dependence". Thus, when we write y=fctn(x) we say that y "depends" on x, and as we have seen, this is the basis of one class of causal notions. Capturing the essence of dependence is a bit of a problem, however, if one wants to speak at an appropriate level of generality. The purpose of this section is to extend the tools of MSC to a general theory of causation based on the idea of dependence.

As always, I assume that there is a set Ω of opportunities. I also continue to assume a collection F, but now this can consist of any functions whatsoever defined on Ω. Before, I referred to these as factors, because they assumed the values 0 or 1, but now I want to allow functions taking values in any sets or mathematical structures whatsoever. In fact, I do not even require that all the elements of F take values in the same set. Thus, some elements of F could be factors, some could be real-valued functions, some could be vector- or matrix-valued functions, and others could take as their values finite groups, digitalized photo-images, or categories of topological spaces. If this seems a little breath-taking, it simply underscores that most of what I will develop here has nothing to do with the scale on which one chooses to make measurements.

Next I want to re-define multiplication. For elements f, g, and h in F, I define their product to be all quantities that can be written as x = fctn(f,g,h). Thus, ΠF now consists of all quantities that can be computed from knowledge of a finite collection from F. In order to distinguish between an element f of F and an element **f** of ΠF, I use the boldface notation, as I have just done.

The $\vee$ operator is defined so that f$\vee$g consists of all quantities that can be written either as fctn(f) or as fctn(g). That is, f$\vee$g is the collection of all quantities that I can compute in the case where I know f, or the case where I know g. Obviously, $\vee\Pi$F is the set of all quantities that can be computed in cases where one of several elements of ΠF is known.

For example, let a, r, d, and c be the area, radius, diameter, and circumference of a circle. Since $a = \pi r^2$ we have a=fctn(π,r) and so a∈ πr. Likewise $a = \pi(d/2)^2$ so a=fctn(π,d) and a∈ πd. Finally, a=cd/4 shows a=fctn(c,d) and a∈ cd. Taken together, these show a∈ cd∨πd∨πr = cd∨(d∨r)π.

Using ∨ in this way may be a little confusing, because it is not how we naturally think of information being packaged (which is one reason why we have trouble thinking about causal pathways). To help, imagine a huge library with a rule that only one book at a time can be checked out. If f and g represent books, then fg represents putting both books together on the table and getting information from them simultaneously. If f and g are only in the huge library, however, then the most you can get is f∨g, because you can only have one of the books at a time.

Returning to our purpose, let y be a function on Ω, again of arbitrary character. I am now ready to say what it means for an f∈ ΠF to be a sufficient cause of y:

f $\overset{s}{\longrightarrow}$ y means that y = fctn(f) is a natural rule

At this point it is critical to say more precisely what I mean by a natural rule. We have already seen that mere functional relationships, even if they are dressed up some, are difficult to use as a definition of causation. Thus, I would like y=fctn(x) to be interpreted to mean that if this equation does not hold, then there is a *natural imperative* to make it hold. This amounts to saying that it is a characteristic of nature to look around at all the causal relationships like y=fctn(x) and to expend effort to make true those that are currently false. What is crucial here is that because I want to think of x as the cause and y as the effect, nature is constrained to make the causal equation true by modifying y, not x. This is the fundamental statement of causal asymmetry.

If we want to go back to an interventionist notion of causation, then assuming that as a causal agent I can set the value of x to whatever I want, and further assuming that the value I choose destroys y=fctn(x), then the causal scenario that plays out is that nature is constrained to modify y to some new value that will satisfy this causal equation. This version of causation provides an explanation for change as nature trying to satisfy all her causal equations.

Continuing to focus on the particular x as a cause of y, the residual cause is defined as

$$b_0 = \vee\{f\in\Pi F_1 : f \dashrightarrow h(y) \text{ for some nontrivial } h\}$$

Saying h is nontrivial here means that it is not constant, so that it measures some aspect of y. Thus b_0 consists of all possible functions one can construct from vectors of elements from F_1 which are sufficient causes of some aspect of y. Recall that F_1 is F with x removed. Sufficient causes of h(y) here are vectors of factors that appear in nontrivial causal equations for h(y). Thus, all possible aspects of y that are involved in causal equations built up from F_1 are in b_0. b_0 is a representation of all the causal aspects of y that are caused by F_1.

The definition of the co-cause of x is

$$b_1 = \vee\{f\in\Pi F_1 : fx \dashrightarrow h(y), f \dashrightarrow h(y) \text{ for some nontrivial } h\}$$

Remember that with our current definition of multiplication fx consists of all functions fctn(f,x). If we define the causes of y in F as

$$C[y|F] = \vee\{f\in\Pi F : f \dashrightarrow h(y) \text{ for some nontrivial } h\}$$

then it is all but obvious that we have the causal equation

$$b_0 \vee b_1 x = C[y|F]$$

We are now in a position to define

$$x \longrightarrow y \text{ means } b_1 \neq \varnothing$$

This means that x is a cause of y if and only if there is some vector f of factors from F_1 such that together with x they appear in a causal equation (in the natural imperative sense) with some aspect of y, but that f is not a sufficient cause of that aspect of y.

It is worthwhile taking stock of where this definition has gotten us. First, it has replaced counterfactual arguments with natural imperative arguments. Although our definition can be used in counterfactual reasoning, there is nothing in the definition itself that uses counterfactuality in any way. If intervening on x invalidates several causal equations, then nature will go about changing whatever needs to be changed to restore them. We need not concern ourselves about the causal

201

equations that do not involve y, when we are trying to define causes of y. This eases some of the problems that we have found with both Rubin's and Pearl's hypothetical response profile approaches, and in fact there does not seem to be any insuperable reason why their profiles could not actually be reinterpreted in the language of natural imperatives.

Secondly, again in contrast to both Rubin's and Pearl's approaches, our definition does not preclude difficulties in establishing causation, or estimating causal effects. Whereas Pearl's approach assumes away most such problems, and Rubin removes problem cases as a matter of definition, our definition allows them.

Thirdly, there is no restriction on the levels of measurement. The basic MSC approach has catapulted us from binary variables, the simplest possible, to the most complex conceivable methods of measurement.

Fourthly, probability plays no role in the definition. This overcomes a very substantial objection to many other causal theories, which depend on probability in a fundamental way. To make these theories plausible, one must imagine that probabilities of events are somehow characteristics of the events themselves. What is true, of course, is that probability only establishes a relationship between the event and the observer, and since different observers can have different objective probabilities for the same event (because they use different sampling schemes, for example), we could have as many causal theories as observers. While there may be elements of subjectivity in any causal theory, this would seem to embrace subjectivity itself as an attractive basic principle.

Fifthly, this notion of dependence includes the usual functional dependence concept, but introduces the idea of *computational pathways*. When I write $f \lor g \overset{\rightarrow}{\rule{0pt}{0pt}} y$ I am asserting that I can compute y from f and then I don't need g, or if I have g I can compute y without f. This is fundamentally different from just saying y=fctn(f,g).

It is perhaps clear that we can now go back and develop the MSC properties of dependence and natural imperative, in analogy to what has been done for binary variables. When b_1 is not empty, we can talk about direct and indirect dependencies. We can introduce sampling from the population of opportunities, and then in specific applications (real-valued variables, for example) work out the conditions that dependence places on the resulting probability models. We can show that dependence has a graphical representation, and that the methods of reversal and double reversal apply. We can do this because we have a well-defined notion of dependence and the MSC tools for studying it.

The notion of natural imperative brings another important aspect to the definition. Under this conception rules are not equations that hold all the time, they are instead equations that nature is compelled to try to satisfy. One can imagine that some of these rules are more important than others, so that nature is willing to expend a great deal of energy satisfying the important ones very rapidly, while the less important ones might be permitted to languish. Anthropomorphisms like this do not explain why nature behaves this way, but they do help us to think about the patterns that we observe. The existence of certain rare elementary particles must be prohibited by fairly strong causal equations, since our best efforts to produce them have such fleeting success. At the other extreme, the forces moving tectonic plates on the Earth's surface are trying to solve equations that became unbalanced millions of years ago.

Perhaps it is fitting to end this section by again referring to Mackie. In his book on causation he characterized it as the *cement* of the universe, that which holds everything together. The concepts of dependence and natural imperative would instead assign to causation the role of the *reason for change* in the universe, that which keeps it forever in motion. Once again, I can end on the note that it is to the credit of the MSC notion, and the ideas that it generates, that one can use it to study versions of causation that span enormously different conceptualizations of what causation really is.

DAG Theory

In developing the MSC approach and the materials for this book, I was well aware, of course, of the modern approach to causation based on *directed acyclic graphs (DAGs)*. Although I believe that there is at a fundamental level a fairly large disconnect between DAG theory and MSC theory, I have been asked multiple times to try to relate the two approaches, and that is the purpose of this section.

First, I call the approach based on directed acyclic graphs "DAG theory" because those who have written on it have not given it a distinctive name (like everyone else, they use "causation" for their notion of causation), and there are too many theoreticians working on the DAG approach to name it after any one of them. In the end, it seems to be the use of DAGs that holds DAG theory together, so the name is natural.

Secondly, I must assume that the reader is familiar with DAG theory, at least at the elementary level, since it is a complex approach, and it would take many pages to explain it in adequate detail. Most of what I will say here is based upon the version in Spirtes, Glymour, and Scheines[1] (SGS), with interpretation and insight from Pearl[2]. Suffice it to say that I do not intend to go very deeply into these impressive works, and that, as I indicated in Section 1, my purpose is not to attack an alternative theory but to illuminate the similarities, and mostly differences, in their approaches.

To begin, a DAG is a finite set of variables, connected by arrows, in such a fashion that you cannot follow the arrows around in a loop. SGS say that each arrow stands for a direct causal relationship between the variable at the tail (the cause) and the variable at the head (the effect). They do not say what causation is, only that arrows in a DAG represent it. In this they are on quite the same footing as MSC; we are both trying to describe how causation works and what its consequences are. In other words, both MSC and DAG are descriptive theories.

SGS justify using a DAG by positing some characteristics of causation. First, no variable causes itself (irreflexivity). Secondly, causation is transitive (if x causes z, and z causes y, then x causes y). Finally, causation is directional (if x causes y, then y cannot cause x). These conditions are sufficient for the existence of a DAG-representation by causal arrows.

Of course the first distinction here is that DAG sees causation as a relationship between variables, whereas MSC sees it as a relationship between factors (that is, event indicators) and therefore between events. MSC tries to extend itself to causation among variables (Section 33), while for DAG it is a simple matter to restrict the theory to little worlds of factors, since a factor is a special kind of variable.

The second distinction is more important, that DAG takes its three rules as axiomatic of a causal system, whereas MSC does not. Under nontrivial implication, for example, a factor can cause itself. Although I regard that as being a little silly, I'm not sure the rest of the theory is harmed by allowing some silly cases. Recall that a sufficient causation only implies nontrivial implication, so that MSC certainly allows irreflexive sufficient causations, if one wants. With respect to transitivity, I have argued that *sufficient* MSC causations should have it, but not causation in general. This is a fundamental distinction. With respect to directionality, I have not given any examples of mutual causation, but I do not believe that MSC theory prohibits them.

Speaking entirely mathematically, the only thing a DAG specifies is a *strict partial order* of the variables. (A strict partial order is a relation that is irreflexive, transitive, and directional. If every pair of variables is ordered, then it is a *total order*, and otherwise there are some for which no ordering can be determined.) A strict partial order can be considered to be the free union of all the total orders that are consistent with it. In other words, if you give me a strict partial order, I should be able to find all the total orders that do not contradict it (that is, for all pairs where we both declare an order, we agree), and conversely, if I give you a collection of total orders, and you find all the ordered pairs that are common to all of them, then you have a strict partial order.

The next set of ideas in DAG theory is to relate properties of a joint probability distribution over all of the variables in the DAG to causal ideas. I contend that, like other causalists, the DAG theorists do not often ground their notion of probability. I think, however, it is likely that they casually assume some kind of random sampling, without saying so. Since this kind of error is fixable, I will not dwell on it. I will remark, however, that the MSC approach develops many of its results without the necessity of any probability. This is again a fundamental distinction, that DAG theory *requires* some underlying probability measure for its basic definitions.

If we go back to the fundamental chain rule of probability, we find that it uses a total order. Given a causal DAG, I can pick any total order consistent with the partial order of the DAG and use the chain rule on that total order to factor the joint probability distribution of all the variables. This means that each component of the product I produce will be of the form pr(x| predecessors of x), where the set of "predecessors of x" depends on which total order I selected, and is in any case just those that precede x in that total order. It is a bed-rock assumption of DAG theory that when I do this, I can drop from "predecessors of x" all variables except those that are "immediate predecessors of x", that is, all those except the ones that are connected directly to x by a causal arrow (and not just by a chain of causal arrows). It is the assumption that I can do this that connects the probability distribution with the DAG.

DAG theorists will be howling at this point, because this is not how they connect a probability distribution with a DAG. It is true, however, and is proved in SGS, that the definition they make implies the one I have just given. The above definition is easier to see, however. Saying that

pr(x|predecessors of x) = pr(x|immediate predecessors of x)

just means that probabilistically x is conditionally independent of its distant predecessors given its immediate predecessors. This uncovers one of the true characterizations of DAG-theory causation. Indirect causal relationships (those of distant predecessors) can be conditioned out using direct causal relationships (immediate predecessors). This specific probabilistic definition underlies all probability-based definitions of causation that I know about. As I showed in Section 19, unless the model is correctly specified, in MSC theory this definition need not hold.

And this leads to perhaps the most immense difference between the MSC and DAG theories. I would claim that except perhaps in rather rare circumstances, DAG theorists assume that all of the causally relevant variables appear in the DAG. Any exogenous variables (those with only out-pointing arrows) are assumed mutually independent of each other. This is so that no causal influences happening outside the DAG will have probabilistic effects inside the DAG. Everything causal has been accounted for in the DAG, so that it is a causally-isolated system, and this explains why the exogenous variables behave like just so much random noise.

At this point, I think it is possible to see why seeking connections between DAG and MSC is likely to become increasingly less useful, the further one goes. This is because DAG assumes that you know all causally relevant relationships, and its definitions depend on this being true. A submodel of a DAG causal model need not be a DAG causal model, because it might have left out something crucial. DAG causation is top-down; you know how everything works, and so you can look at how particular things work. MSC is bottom-up, or more positively, constructivist. You try to work with overly-simple systems that you can actually observe, being aware of the threats to the validity of your work, and you expand your scope as you discover the problems.

(For purists, I will say that in addition to the above conditional independence condition, there is a further condition. Each x must be conditionally independent of all unrelated variables (those that neither precede nor follow x), given its predecessors. If these two conditional independence conditions hold for every x in the graph, then the probability distribution is paired with the graph. The collection of conditional independencies exhibited by all probability distributions that are paired with a given graph are said to be implied by the graph. A particular probability distribution paired with the graph is *faithful* to the graph if it exhibits those and only those conditional independencies that are implied by the graph. SGS seem to take genuine cases of causation to be those represented by a DAG and a faithful, paired probability distribution.)

In all of this, it may seem that DAG theory is nothing more than an elaborate theory of representing independence and conditional independence. The only connections with actual causation seems to be (1) the arrows are declared to represent direct causal relationships, and (2) indirect causal relationships are represented by conditional independence conditions. While these connections might be seen as being appropriate for a purely descriptive theory, Pearl goes one step further, in order to provide an operational definition of cause. He says that we should first write down the factorization of the joint probability distribution that is implied by the DAG. This is a product of conditional probability distributions of each of the variables, given all its immediate predecessors in the strict partial order of the DAG. Now select two variables, x and y, and ask whether x causes y. To get the answer, (1) strike the conditional probability distribution of x from the product, and (2) everywhere x occurs in a conditional distribution (which will always be "behind the bar"), insert the value that you intend to set x equal to. Pearl then says that the joint probability distribution that you produce with these two steps represents the correct probabilities for the situation in which you override all causes of x in the DAG, set x equal to your intended value, while not disturbing any of the other causal patterns in the DAG. Integrate out all variables except y, leaving you with either (1) a marginal distribution for y, in which case x is not a cause of y, or (2) a conditional probability distribution for y which depends on x, in which case x is a cause of y.

This is not the place to debate the virtues and drawbacks of Pearl's definition. I will restrict my comments to the relationship between DAG causation (in the Pearl version, or the earlier SGS version, either one) and MSC. The most you can hope for in the DAG/Pearl theory is one or more conditional probability distributions (in the usual sense, or in Pearl's sense of setting x) that are said to embody causal facts. I have not found the notion of *sufficiency* to play much if any role in this theory, and since this is the starting point of MSC, there are clearly difficulties in forming a connection. I would imagine that (restricting consideration to factors) $pr(y=1|x_1=1,x_2=1,...,x_k=1) = 1$ might count as sufficiency in the DAG/Pearl sense. (Presumably we would extend Pearl's notion of setting a single variable to setting a collection $x_1,...,x_k$ of variables, and indeed just such an operation is given in SGS.) It seems to me plausible, however, that in an entire DAG no such relationship would ever occur, leaving no cases of sufficiency, and therefore no connection point with MSC.

It this were the case (and it seems to be in virtually all examples), then one needs to go back again to the question of what probability means in the DAG theory. If $pr(y=1|x_1=1,x_2=1,...,x_k=1)<1$ in all cases, then one interpretation is that there are other factors that go into the determination of y, but they are occult to us, and so probability is a reasonable language for talking about what we are restricted to see. I realize that there are other interpretations of probability, but this one seems particularly natural in the context of discussions about causation. If this is the right approach, then SGS do not require these extra latent factors to be present in the DAG. Indeed, if one were to require this, one would be taking an enormous step toward specifying the causal field, along the lines that I have done in developing MSC theory. Thus, although there is the theoretical possibility of a connection here, empirically it does not seem to be salient, in the sense that few if any DAGs specify the causal field to the point that causal relations are deterministic; indeed, given the way the DAG theory is constructed, it is hard to imagine what that would mean.

A consequence of this is that DAG theory does not specify causal patterns at the same level of detail that MSC does. In a sense, DAG theory is coarser (or more positively, higher-level) than MSC. SGS note this in their book, where they point out that nothing in the DAG will exhibit the details of how the variables relate to each other. In my words, DAGs cannot exhibit phenomena such a dual causation or paradoxical causation, and do not even provide an adequate language for talking about causal pathways. One of the reasons that I have developed MSC graphics the way I did was to overcome this deficiency.

To summarize, although it does not seem impossible to use DAG/Pearl causation as one that could feed into the MSC constructivist program, there are some significant problems to overcome. The DAG approach does not provide a sufficiently rich language for talking about causal pathways. It also is based quite considerably on a probability distribution that is connected to the causal structure, so that one might have no instances of sufficiency with which to start the MSC process. Pearl's definition of a new kind of conditioning, based on a minimal intervention that changes only specified variables and nothing else, seems to have understandable properties only at the high-level of language that is used in DAGs. Whether his "setting" operation can be defined meaningfully in the MSC setting remains a question.

Finally, DAG is a top-down theory, while MSC is a bottom-up theory. It is, perhaps, true that Nature designed causation in our part of the universe based on a huge DAG. But as humble human scientists, I think we have to try to understand it constructively, and that is what MSC does.

References

1. Spirtes P, Glymour C, Scheines R. Causation, Prediction, and Search. Lecture Notes in Statistics 81. New York: Springer Verlag, 1993
2. Pearl J. Causality. Cambridge UK: Cambridge University Press, 2000.

Epilogue

If it turns out, for the remainder of the time that humans have in this universe, that philosophers do not advance the philosophy of causation beyond where it is today, this may mean rather little, either for the humdrum daily life of humanity or for the discipline of philosophy. This would be true because most people have a commonsense notion of causation that serves them perfectly well in their ordinary lives (suggesting that Hume's skepticism was perhaps too pessimistic). They know nothing of the philosophical issues, nor do they need to know them. It would also be true because in our current era philosophers are often permitted to go their own ways, without having the excessive baggage of connection to the world of action. They may know rather little of the world of science, nor do they need to know it.

I am not so sanguine, however, about our prospects in biomedical science, where I work, if we do not make more progress in conceiving our problems in causal terms. The cosmologist John Barrow has suggested a particularly dim possible future, in which the expansion of scientific questions overwhelms society's willingness or ability to pay for work on them, with the result that less and less useful science will actually be done.

We do not have to wait for Barrow's speculation to happen before being concerned. We can already see rather large amounts of money spent on research that contributes only very tangentially to causal understanding. For example, in the study of disease nowadays data presentations are nearly always in the form shown in Figure 1. There are column headings for the two disease outcomes, and then a series of pairs of lines in which one of the putative causes assumes its 0 or 1 value. The remainder of the display is almost universally taken up by odds ratios and the accompanying statistical impedimenta. This display is, of course, equivalent to the causal model(s) shown in Figure 2. I hope that the reader who has progressed this far will have no difficulty understanding how completely inadequate these causal models are.

If the minimal sufficient cause approach is anything like the truth, then we are spending enormous sums in order to do research that is severely diminished in its ability to inform us about fundamental causal processes. We are doing this in part because the dead hand of conventionality compels researchers to put their results into the primitive form of Figure 1 in order to get published. The editors and referees of our scientific journals are the minions of oblivion who enforce this mindless uniformity.

Factor		Diseased	Not Diseased	Odds Ratio	Confidence Interval
A	0	#	#		
	1	#	#	#	#
B	0	#	#		
	1	#	#	#	#
C	0	#	#		
	1	#	#	#	#

Figure 1. Conventional presentation of factors and disease.

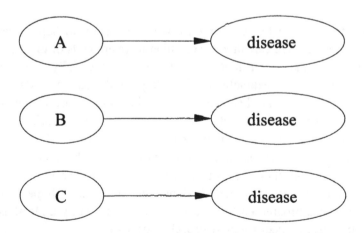

Figure 2. Causal model implied by the data presentation of Figure 1.

One might argue, of course, that the reason causal analysis does not make more impact on biomedical science is that we often do not have good causal hypotheses. There are two reasons to be suspicious of this argument. The first is that following David Hume's withering 18th century critique of causation, scientists have been extremely tentative about using the "C-word", and have consequently made far less of an attempt to develop causal hypotheses than if Hume had directed his skepticism elsewhere. (As I have noted, we may observe that the calculus as developed by Newton and Leibniz has at least as many philosophical holes as causation does; if Hume had attacked those, leaving causation alone, and scientists had reacted similarly, we would today be missing huge pieces of mathematics that we have relied on for progress.)

But there is an even more telling fact about the lowly state of causation in the modern era. Even when causal schemas are put forward, usually in editorials or "opinion pieces", and even when these could be translated into causal models for analysis, one searches in vain for research designs based on the causal models, or for data analyses using any causal principles. So the fact is that even when we do have some vision of what the causal picture is for a certain disease, we do not organize and analyze our research according to that vision.

In the pages above I have argued that a causal diagram is related to a probability model, and it is then obvious that the latter can be used for analysis. The causal arrows change to conditional probability distribution arrows, although sometimes the diagram must be processed, using techniques such as reversal or double reversal. Nonetheless, the start is a causal diagram from which a probability diagram can be derived. Despite the simplicity of this idea, it is not being used. I have seen too many grant proposals submitted to the National Institutes of Health in which, if you graph out the causal model that the investigators clearly had in mind as they designed the application, and then you set it next to the plan they propose for analyzing the data, there is simply no correspondence. Astonishingly, this lack of correspondence appears to be almost completely irrelevant to whether the application is funded.

I would argue that one consequence of our inadequate training in thinking about causation is our general inability to produce good causal

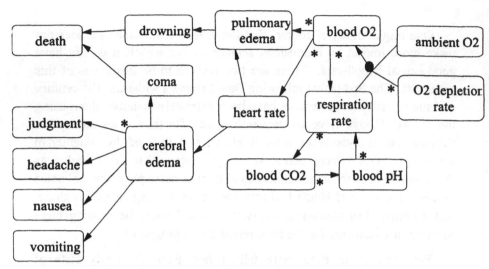

Figure 3. Causal diagram for mountain sickness (Houston CS. Mountain sickness. *Scientific American* (Special Issue on Medicine) 1993;150-155). All residual causes and co-causes are omitted for clarity.

diagrams. When I first began considering these issues I questioned whether the creation of a causal diagram was really possible for most diseases, irrespective of whether it would be useful. I went to various literatures where there were overviews of disease processes, and I found it extraordinarily difficult to figure out how to represent the narrative as a diagram. At first this discouraged me about whether causal diagrams were generally possible, but eventually I realized that the task was getting easier as I did more and more of them. The problems were largely in my lack of training.

An example of an early effort is shown in Figure 3. The disease here is mountain sickness. Although we probably have a longer historical record of this than any other disease, it was not until the nineteenth century that it was appreciated that oxygen pressure drops with altitude, and that this is a cause of the disease. As the ambient oxygen concentration goes down, and the oxygen depletion rate rises, in the face of an inadequate respiratory response, blood oxygen levels go down. Falling blood oxygen raises the respiration rate, which feeds back to raise blood oxygen. There is another feedback loop, however, in which increasing respiration lowers blood carbon dioxide, which raises blood pH, which lowers the respiration rate. It is the fact that the respiration rate is locked in two feedback loops that leads to the paradoxical cycles of over-breathing and under-breathing that exist among even the earliest accounts of the disease. As blood oxygen goes down, pulmonary edema sets in, both due to a direct effect and also due to an indirect effect that blood oxygen has on the heart rate. The increased heart rate also stimulates cerebral edema, which gives rise to the common but non-threatening symptoms of the disease (such as impaired judgment), but can also lead to coma and to death. Another pathway to death is through pulmonary edema leading to drowning in one's own lung fluid.

I think it is remarkable how much easier it is to see what the causal relationships are from the diagram than it is from the narrative. Moreover, from the diagram we can imagine experiments that could test each part of the diagram. Finally, we have a much deeper appreciation of the disease process, and what a reasonable treatment might consist of, than if our causal picture were "a too rapid ascent causes mountain sickness".

In the absence of any college courses to improve our general graphical abilities, I would recommend a book by de Bono[1]. This book probably belongs in the "business, self-help" section, but it rises above its origins by encouraging us to use our natural abilities to think in terms of abstract concepts, and to see connections among them, in constructing "first draft" versions of the bubbles-and-arrows graphs like Figure 3. It helps us to be open, free, and creative in thinking about relationships that may be causal. After following de Bono, the second step is to submit the resulting graphics to criticism, and empirical test in the real world. For the most part, this book has been about the second part, but the first part is important, too.

Minimal sufficient cause is not the only approach that can be taken to thinking about causation, nor should it be. We understand little enough about causation to be failing to use any reasonable approach that sheds light on conceptualization and analysis. It has not been my purpose in writing this book to try to rule out causal theories because they disagree with MSC, but rather to make two related points. First, it is possible to discuss, debate, and understand properties that causation ought to have, even before we have a firm, unequivocal definition of causation. Secondly, it is necessary to develop causal theories in such a fashion that they can be meaningfully compared to each other, otherwise they will lie forever beyond the realm of science. It is my hope that this book will help to advance thinking and discussion about all approaches to causation.

Reference

1. de Bono E. Water Logic: The Alternative to I am Right and You are Wrong. London UK, Viking, 1993

Further Reading

The literature on causation is enormous, while the literature on MSC is tiny. In this section I would like to emphasize those few MSC references, and point out some additional readings on approaches to causation that are relevant to MSC issues. There is no pretense to completeness, and the remarks are admittedly subjective.

Mackie JL. Causes and conditions. *American Philosophical Quarterly* 1965 Oct;2/4:245-255. (Reproduced in part in Sosa E, Tooley M. (eds.) Causation. Oxford: Oxford University Press, 1993)

Although Mackie alludes to earlier work, this is the source article for the minimal sufficient cause approach. He gives a remarkably clear account this new conditional equivalence viewpoint, and the problems it solves. Even for those who do not like to read philosophy, this is a worthwhile article.

Rothman KJ. Causes. *American Journal of Epidemiology* 1976;104:587-592. (Reproduced in Rothman KJ. (ed.) Causal Inference. Chestnut Hill MA: Epidemiology Resources, 1988)

Here we find the definition of sufficient pathways and minimal sufficient causes. This article is quite clear about how these concepts should be defined and what role they should play in epidemiology. Rothman also wanted to account for antagonism and synergy among causes, but in the absence of a firm logical base, this is not the best part of the article.

As an aside, the Causal Inference volume contains a contribution from a philosopher, the reactions of the epidemiologists, and then re-reactions of the philosopher, which provide a fascinating picture of how these two disciplines talk past each other, and indicates how very rarely they ever come into contact.

Sheps MC. Shall we count the living or the dead? *New England Journal of Medicine* 1958;259:1210-1214

In this and the other two articles cited at the end of Section 8, Sheps put forward her measure of excess occurrence. Statisticians tend to evaluate effect measures in terms of their statistical or esthetic properties, and so Sheps' measure did not flourish. Her articles are well worth reading.

Spirtes P, Glymour C, Scheines R. Causation, Prediction, and Search. Lecture Notes in Statistics 81. New York: Springer Verlag, 1993

McKim VR, Turner SP. (eds) Causality in Crisis? Notre Dame IN, University of Notre Dame Press, 1997

The first of these is *must* reading for anyone who wants a complete understanding of modern causal diagrams. It is a rather long volume, and written much in the mathematical style, but it contains the fundamental definitions and arguments for thinking about causation in terms of directed acyclic graphs (DAG). It is important to realize that this is a very general approach, and that it includes as special cases all of the causal graphs of the social sciences.

The second volume is a collection on several issues, but a number of the articles are dedicated to discussions of the previous book. There are good, simplified versions of the DAG approach, and one rousing piece in opposition by statistician David Freedman.

Pearl J. Causal diagrams for empirical research. Biometrika 1995;82:669-710

In this article Judea Pearl advanced the idea that a DAG is causal in the sense that (and presumably only if) when we control one of its variables, the probability distribution over the remainder can be obtained by dividing out the conditional distribution of the controlled factor, and setting all remaining occurrences of it to the control value. It could be argued that this interpretation is the missing piece in the Spirtes, Glymour and Scheines volume.

Pearl J. Causality. Cambridge UK: Cambridge Univ Press, 2000

More than ten years of research by Pearl and his colleagues is collected together, and articulated with new examples, insights, and arguments. At the moment, this is the definitive volume for understanding the DAG approach to causation, in the Pearl version.

Heckerman D, Shacter R. Decision-theoretic foundations for causal reasoning. Journal of Artificial Intelligence Research 1995;3:405-430

This can be considered an elaboration of both the counterfactual approach and Pearl's approach. "Decisions" are factors that can (in some unspecified way) be controlled by investigators, and the only other thing necessary to describe the model is the "state of the world", meaning all factors not influenced by "decisions". Factor x causes factor y if x depends on the state of the world and the decisions, and y depends only on the state of the world and x. Due to the rather idiosyncratic use of "state of the world", this approach is in fact a mathematical system for talking in detail about counterfactual arguments. Whether its definition of cause goes beyond Rubin is questionable.

Robins J. Causal inference from complex longitudinal data. In Berkane (ed). Latent Variable Modeling and Applications to Causality. Lecture Notes in Statistics 120. New York: Springer Verlag, 1997:69-118

Robins uses Rubin's hypothetical response profile and the DAG method of representing causal probability distributions to deduce how one should analyze certain kinds of longitudinal studies. Although this particular article suffers from some infelicitous notation, it is well worth plowing through for its insights.

Holland PW. Statistics and causal inference. Journal of the American Statistical Association 1986;81:945-960

This is a very clear exposition of Rubin's hypothetical profile method, including some partisan argument in its favor. Part of why it is worth reading is that Rubin is virtually the only statistician to have put forward a coherent argument for causal analysis, and to press his colleagues (with little perceptible success) to adopt it. Regardless how one views the approach, it contributes valuable insights into how probability models can go wrong in causal situations.

Weinberg CR.   Applicability of the simple independent action model to epidemiologic studies involving two factors and a dichotomous outcome. *American Journal of Epidemiology* 1986;123:162-173

Here is a derivation of the two-factor causal model (probability version), from the standpoint of toxicology, without any discussion of causal theory.

Shafer G. The Art of Causal Conjecture. Cambridge MA: The MIT Press. 1996

The basic tool of this approach is the event-tree, which is a way of representing both transitions from one state to another, as well as complete pathways involving multiple transitions. Although the earlier part of the book is rather thick with definitions, not always sufficiently motivated, in general Shafer is exceedingly clear about his arguments. Ultimately, causation is viewed as probability-raising, but in the event-tree context this a more powerful operation than in Patrick Suppes classical monograph.

Index